STRONGER TOGETHER

Starting a Health Team
in Your Congregation

STRONGER TOGETHER

Starting a Health Team in Your Congregation

JILL WESTBERG MCNAMARA

Published on the occasion of the 27th Annual Westberg Symposium

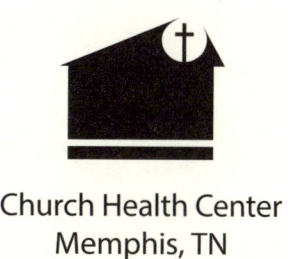

Church Health Center
Memphis, TN

About the Church Health Center

The Church Health Center seeks to reclaim the church's biblical commitment to care for our bodies and our spirits. The Center's ministries provide health care for the working uninsured and promote healthy bodies and spirits for all. To learn more about the Center, visit www.ChurchHealthCenter.org. To learn more about our magazine on health ministry, *Church Health Reader*, visit www.chreader.org.

Stronger Together: Starting a Health Team in Your Congregation
Part 1 © 2014 Jill Westberg McNamara
Part 2 © 2014 Church Health Center

ISBN: 978-1-62144-041-3

Printed in the United States of America

The Church Health Center is proud to publish this resource using recycled materials.

Written by Jill Westberg McNamara
Edited by Susan Martins Miller, John Shorb, and Stacy Smith
Cover Design by Rachel Thompson Davis
Layout and design by Rachel Thompson Davis and Lizy Heard

The Church Health Center welcomes your feedback. Please send your comments to FCO@churchhealthcenter.org.

To my father, Granger E. Westberg.
His passion for faith communities and health lives on.

Contents

May God bless you with *discomfort* … at easy answers, half-truths and superficial relationships so that you may live deep within your heart.

May God bless you with *anger* … at injustice, oppression and exploitation of people so that you may work for justice, freedom, and peace.

May God bless you with *tears* … to shed for those who suffer from pain, rejection, starvation and war so that you may reach out your hand to comfort them and turn their pain into joy.

And may God bless you with enough *foolishness* … to believe that you can make a difference in this world, so that you can do what others claim cannot be done.

Imagine a congregation that exemplifies this Franciscan benediction.

Each moment would be vital, and people would listen fully with their hearts.

Lively discussions and questions would prevail.

Because everyone would foolishly believe they could make a difference, the world would be transformed.

Please Read This First

I've written this section because, if like me, you rarely read nonfiction from beginning to end, you might get a bit confused regarding a few points. Hopefully I caught your attention before you started scratching your head.

A Note on Faith Community Nursing

If you picked up this book because you want to have or be a faith community nurse, you're on the right track. Over time we have learned that having a health team to precede and to support the nurse makes for a stronger and longer lasting health ministry. In Part 2, you will find information on faith community nurses as well as recommendations for other resources.

A Note on Religious Diversity

This book focuses mainly on Christian congregations starting health teams, yet religious groups and people across the world are active in health and wellness. In certain areas, Native Americans are incorporating their spirituality into western medicine. Muslims are networking with Christian communities and public health agencies to address mental illness. Faith community nurses serve in synagogues, mosques and temples all over the world. It is important to remember that though this is a book from the Christian perspective, health ministry occurs in various ways in all religious traditions.

A Note on Language

Even though I use *congregation* instead of *church* to be more inclusive, this book reflects the Christian perspective. However, because every major faith has a mandate to care for others, this book should still be applicable to any faith community. When you get to certain parts, though, like justifying a health team to your congregation, you will obviously need to draw from your own tradition.

To return to faith community nurses, I want to assure you that, yes, it is the same as a parish nurse. The name has changed because we want to include all faiths and because the American Nurses Association determined this name as the general term. Occasionally the term parish nurse will surface in this writing, especially if I am referring to something in the past or I am quoting someone else.

Preface

A Guiding Headlight

"How often the church has been an echo rather than a voice, a taillight behind the Supreme Court and other secular agencies, rather than a headlight guiding men progressively and decisively to higher levels of understanding."
—Rev. Dr. Martin Luther King, Jr.[1]

As a young girl, I had no clue that Jesus was a radical. My Christian beliefs were based on a medley of images sanitized for children—gentle lambs strolling with Jesus—hymns that dragged, Scriptures like, "Let the little children come unto me," and noodle casseroles. Where was the energy? The vision? The controversy?

The Jesus I learned about as a child was, frankly, a bit of a wimp. In the largely white, middle-class churches our family belonged to, politeness and conformity presided. I was probably 19 before it hit me that Jesus was anything but well behaved.

Jesus was, in fact, all about rocking the boat. Jesus argued with the religious authorities and hung out with tax collectors. He listened to women. He reached out and touched people with disabilities, a major taboo of his time. He cared about children, another line-crossing for his time. He was a reformer. He was a radical. He loved people as they came to him. His actions had nothing to do with good manners.

Too often congregations have become like museums and clubs, with walls built up for protection rather than welcome. We dress in our Sunday finery and put on our best manners. Asked how we are, the response is "fine" or "everything's wonderful." We are covering up our authentic selves—who we are deep inside. We don't expose our brokenness for fear of rejection, out of concern about what others think. Little change can take place in this type of atmosphere.

We need to rock the boat. The health care system in the United States needs to be shaken. We have nearly come to accept an obesity epidemic that results in multiple medical issues. Millions of people are still without health insurance. Medication is used at astoundingly high levels. Poverty levels have only grown. No doubt, you know about these challenges and more.

We need to risk speaking and acting from the depths of our hearts. We need to be that guiding headlight that Martin Luther King, Jr. so prophetically called each one of us to be   that Jesus called each of us to be. We need to do things differently so that we can see improvements in the health of individuals, communities of faith, and communities at large—all of the world.

Stronger Together

Introduction

love this!

"Those who love you are not fooled by mistakes you have made or dark images you hold about yourself. They remember your beauty when you feel ugly; your wholeness when you are broken; your innocence when you feel guilty; and your purpose when you are confused."
—African saying

Thousands of congregations have a registered nurse as part of their ministry team. First, the good news: congregations are reclaiming their role in health care. They are caring for people as they always have, by visiting the homebound, taking meals to the sick, and praying for others. Research indicates that people who attend churches regularly stay healthier than people who rarely or never attend services. Some congregations have health professionals or knowledgeable lay people in their midst.

We are already poised for the work ahead of us. Yet many of us underestimate our capabilities.

Granted, we are limited in terms of how much we can take on, especially those of us whose communities are smaller in size, but what else is holding us back? Are we afraid to dream big? Are we unable to figure out the necessary logistics? Are we too isolated? Are we afraid to rock the boat as Jesus did?

Starting a health team in your congregation offers a strong foundation for addressing the most critical health challenges where you live and in our increasingly connected global community. Congregations can move the needle on huge issues if we put our minds, hands, and feet to work. In 2002, according to the National Center for Health Statistics, the top four causes of death in the United States were heart disease, cancer, stroke, and chronic lower respiratory disease. Leading reasons people develop these diseases include poor diet, tobacco, alcohol, and lack of exercise. If people make changes in each of these areas, they will probably stay healthier. Congregations can encourage and assist people in making those changes.

> Congregations can move the needle on huge issues if we put our minds, hands, and feet to work.

Most of us already know, in this endless age of self-help, how we can become healthier. Magazines, books, and the Internet tell us how to lower cholesterol, how to satisfy our sex lives, and how to deal with anger. Much of this information is right on target. People in the United States, at least those of us who are fairly privileged, should be incredibly healthy.

The problem is, we just don't do it. At least not for long. We get sidetracked or we give up when the results are not as immediate as we'd hoped. I believe congregations can make the difference. They have a continual connection with about half of the population in the United States. If congregations took on any number of health issues, the benefits could be astonishing.

I have been working on health and wellness in congregations since 1979, when a health team was formed at my church, Community of Christ the Servant in Lombard, Illinois. Jack Lundin, the pastor, loved the idea of Wholistic Health Centers,[1] but in our small church, a health center was not feasible. There was neither the space nor the money. Yet Jack felt that churches could be more intentional about health. So he dreamed up what he named the "health cabinet." His logic was that each home has a medicine cabinet so each church should have a health cabinet.

We started five unique projects. We expected to see the projects succeed, but the health team evolved into much more than the projects. The team's influence on the entire congregation became a major thrust. It acted as a catalyst, encouraging people and the existing committees to keep in mind elements such as caring and purpose as they carried out their ministries.

The response at Community of Christ the Servant was so enthusiastic that, with the help of a grant from the Wheat Ridge Foundation, I asked four other churches in the Chicago area to become pilots (First Congregational Church in Downers Grove; Ascension Lutheran Church in Riverside; Augustana Lutheran Church in Chicago; Marley Community Church in Marley). Each church had different qualities, so the model that resulted from these pilots was flexible, allowing for uniqueness.

A few years later, I began work at the Evangelical Hospital Association (now Advocate Health Care in the Chicago area) to encourage the churches connected with its five hospitals to do more with their health ministries. After the enthusiasm expressed by the five pilot churches, I thought my job would be a snap. It wasn't. Although I probably spoke with over one hundred churches, few expressed long-term interest. It was a worthy concept, but in most churches, people were too busy to add one more committee. I tried approaching churches through many avenues including a newsletter and the social work department at Good Samaritan Hospital. This helped, but not enough. I tried to find other groups or individuals who could give me advice and support, but few people in the country were attempting what I was doing. After three years, I resigned. But the seed had been planted.

Over the next 19 years I worked in other fields, but people, including my father, persevered. More hospitals hired people to do outreach to congregations. The parish nurse, now called the faith community nurse, took form. In fact, it was because of the faith community nurses that congregations began to see the importance of a health team. So, in 2002, when I received a call from a chaplain at Good Samaritan Hospital in Downer's Grove, Illinois, it was to ask me to speak about health teams. After a great deal of skepticism my interest was rekindled.

> "The major agency to support health and healing is the local congregation."[2]
>
> —Rev. Martin Marty, Fairfax M. Cone Distinguished Service Professor Emeritus of the History of Modern Christianity, University of Chicago

In this book, I am excited to present years of learning since those initial days. I have discussed health ministry with people from all over the country (and a few outside of the United States) who pursued the dream of health ministry. Their ministries took many forms. My hope is that by using this book you will be able to shape a health ministry that is a right fit for your situation.

Today, I see the concept of a team as the most effective approach for health and wellness in congregations.

The strength of a team approach includes:

- A team assumes a group of people; you are much stronger working together!
- A team requires action and innovation. A team is not satisfied with doing things "the way we've always done them."
- A team might assemble for a time-limited project or it might live on for years to do many projects.
- A team's structure is flexible according to what works in your situation. It might be structured like a committee or it might be quite informal.

In this book, I have paired each phase of creating a health team with a story. I see narrative as key to making this work come to life. You will find the foundational elements to building an effective health team in your congregation alongside real-life inspiration and theological grounding. Logistics and tips are wonderful, and I have shared them throughout the book. But nothing beats a solid foundation. It is important to take your time in learning about faith and health to develop the strong roots that will lead to a long-lasting vision for your congregation.

We might not realize it, but as people of faith we are already prepared for the work ahead of us. We have the theological grounding. We have the mandate from Jesus to go "preach the kingdom of God and heal the sick." In our midst there are healers, dreamers, doers, organizers, and thinkers who can make almost anything happen. It's a matter of taking those first steps to work together toward becoming that guiding headlight. The challenges before us are immense. Yet we have the faith that we are in the world to bring God's love and justice to all people, one step at a time.

PART 1
Starting Your Health Team

1
Building Foundations:
What motivates your health team?

"Thus from the outset the ministry of healing was considered to be as integral a part of the church's work as the ministry of Word or Sacrament with which it is fundamentally linked."
—Phyllis L. Garlick, *Man's Search for Health*[1]

Why are you holding this book?

If others are looking over your shoulder, what brings them there? What motivates you to dream of a health team in your congregation?

It's crucial to make sure you've thought through the foundational aspects of your purpose together. Mary Chase-Ziolek, professor of health ministries and nursing at North Park University, offers this advice: "When you try to engage congregations in promoting health, you need to start with the question: how does health fit with our tradition and our beliefs? In the case of Christianity, what does our Scripture have to say? What does our religious tradition have to say about how health fits in to the life of a church?"[2] In that spirit, I want to begin this step with a glimpse into the possibilities of Scripture, for health and wellness and also for health teams as a concept rooted in the Bible.

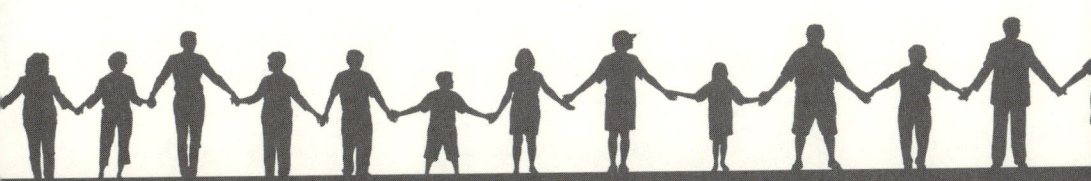

In this chapter, we will:
- **Examine** Jesus' model for healing
- **Define** health
- **Define** team

The Model of Jesus and His Disciples for Healing

Jesus sent his disciples—a group of people he chose and assembled—out to do and eventually continue his ministry. He told them to preach the kingdom of God and heal the sick. Jesus' ministry stressed healing the whole person. As was natural in his Hebrew tradition, he did not separate the body from the mind and the spirit. He was always concerned about healing a person whose body showed signs of illness, but he also paid close attention to other manifestations of illness in the person's life.

Jesus dealt with relationships within people, between people and God, between people and their neighbors, and between people and the world. These relationships gave a necessary perspective to the picture and allowed healing to be approached in a wholistic way.

The book of Acts records how well the early church carried out this commission, caring for whole persons and not just spirits or bodies. Phyllis L. Garlick, author of *Man's Search for Health*, writes: "They were inspired by a sense of wholeness in their mission to the world. They believed that the new quality of life, which Christ came to impart, was to extend to the whole of man's being, body, soul, and spirit. Thus from the outset the ministry of healing was considered to be as integral a part of the church's work as the ministry of Word or Sacrament with which it is fundamentally linked."[4]

Mark 2:1–12 illustrates how Jesus' healings included both the physical and the spiritual realms. In the first verses, when a paralyzed man was brought to Jesus, he said simply, "My child, your sins are forgiven." In doing so he went beyond the man's physical ills to touch the deeper causes of the paralysis. The man took up his pallet and walked because Jesus understood that the body and spirit are a unity.

Jesus' ministry emphasized empowering other people to do healing work. Jesus was a teacher and also, in today's lingo, a team leader. He gathered his

> "Jesus calls all who follow him to demonstrate the same priority of healing the whole person ... If we're going to do what Jesus did, and as his first-century followers did, we must find some way to be involved in a ministry of healing."[3]
>
> —G. Scott Morris, founder and CEO of the Church Health Center

disciples to spread the word and to help him accomplish his ministry on earth. It took a team to lower the man through the roof of the house (Mark 2:4). Jesus modeled for us that we are to go forth, assemble a team, and heal people.

Defining Health

The discoveries, the procedures, and the medicines of medical science are truly amazing. Indeed, much has occurred since Jesus walked among us. Yet as Jesus' ministry demonstrates and as current studies point out, the biomedical model contains only part of the answer. We need to take a wholistic approach that takes into account people's attitudes, environments, and relationships. How might each of these dimensions affect our physical, spiritual, or emotional health?

In their book, *Dust and Breath: Faith, Health, and Why the Church Should Care about Both*, Kendra Hotz and Matthew Mathews write: "Good health allows us to live out our God-given identities. … Comprehensive healthcare, therefore, must seek not only to remove disease but also to create conditions and structures that allow for holistic health."[6] The healthier our body, mind, and spirit are, the more effectively we can live out who God intends us to be.

It is explicitly the work of congregations to attend to everything from safety in our larger communities to visiting us at the end of our lives. We are active agents in the creation of community and the building up of families.

> "And in spite of its best efforts to domesticate Jesus, the Church knows and frequently fears that his message will be rediscovered."[5]
>
> —*William Sloane Coffin, senior minister of Riverside Church, New York City, 1977–1987, author of* The Courage to Love

Often congregations are literally at the crossroads of communities, whether in small towns or major urban centers. When people are in pain or suffering loss, they often find their way to congregations. We can and do make a major difference in this work.

The Institute of Medicine also sees health in a more inclusive way, defining health as "the state of well-being and the capability to function in the face of changing circumstances."[7] Pay attention to the term *changing circumstances*. At a core individual level, we continually encounter change. Some of the changes, like getting married or starting a higher-level job, can be positive (though not always). Other changes can be negative—for instance, the death

---

RECOMMENDED READING

Educating ourselves about faith and health is a part of the process at all points. Reading the following books will provide a great foundation.

On the roots and theology of health ministry:
Dust and Breath: Faith and Health and Why the Church Should Care about Both by Kendra Hotz and Matthew Mathews
God, Health, and Happiness: Discover Wholeness in Body and Spirit by G. Scott Morris
Deeply Woven Roots: Improving the Quality of Life in Your Community by Gary Gunderson
The Healing Word: Preaching and Teaching Health Ministry by Deborah Patterson
Health, Healing and the Church's Mission: Biblical Perspectives and Moral Priorities by William M. Swartley
Health, Healing, & Wholeness: Engaging Congregations in Ministries of Health by Mary Chase-Ziolek

On health care and spirituality:
A Balm for Gilead: Meditations on Spirituality and the Healing Arts by Daniel P. Sulmasy
Medicine as Ministry: Reflections on Suffering, Ethics, and Hope by Margaret E. Mohrmann
Reclaiming the Body: Christians and the Faithful Use of Modern Medicine by Joel Shuman and Brian Volck
Paging God: Religion in the Halls of Medicine by Wendy Cadge

On church history:
Healing in the History of Christianity by Amanda Porterfield
Healing and Christianity by Morton Kelsey
Medicine and Health Care in Early Christianity by Gary B. Ferngren

of a loved one, financial problems, or destruction due to a natural disaster. All changes, both positive and negative, cause stress. The greater our level of stress, the more likely we are to get sick.

Our ability to deal with stress depends on how well we can adapt to new situations. Adaptability is linked to our spirits. Do we have the faith, the grounding, to believe we can make it through? Do our lives have enough meaning to make it worth the struggle? Are we able to lessen some of the anxiety by trusting in God? Are we able to draw on the strength within us?

Where is our congregation in this mix? Is there a presence from the congregation at my hospital bedside? Am I active in service to others? What kind of structure and support are we building at the community level for people to thrive?

This concept of thriving is important for our work to create health teams. We know now that health is much more than the absence of disease. For true health, we want people to thrive and not simply survive. We need to consider the strengths of the whole person, not just the absence of weaknesses.

When we envision health as more than the absence of disease, health becomes empowering. Health allows us to respond to the call of God, to act on possibilities that are open to us and lead toward fulfillment.

Every congregation has the potential to help make each person's days become full of life and love, despite all the hesitancy and resistance. The spiritual component is key here: congregations can motivate people at a level not tapped by most institutions. But the most pressing question persists: how can a congregation have the courage and the imagination to lead the way?

Defining Team

Health teams are the enabling factor for congregations to act nimbly and effectively to address health and wellness issues. The role of health teams is vital to accomplishing the Scriptural mandate: preach the kingdom of God and heal the sick. Complex health challenges certainly cannot be met by any one person within a congregation, even if that person is a full time staff member.

But what is a team? This seems like a simple question, but we all come to the question with various backgrounds.

Teams offer a flexible alternative to institutional mainstays, but if you're not careful they can quickly become stale and purposeless like any other group. Teams are action oriented. They continually try out fresh approaches to reach goals. They can be long-term, like a committee, or short-term, like a task force. Regardless of its duration a health team will always look to improve the health ministry.

Teams can come in all forms and sizes. For some, the word *team* might primarily indicate something like a sports team, a drill team, or a project team. Yet teams are distinct from groups. A team has a purpose while members of a group might have something in common yet no purpose (such as fans of a certain film or book). In some congregational structures, a team may be established with an umbrella of responsibilities and connection to leadership, while in others a team is a small group of people who want to nimbly respond to a need while enjoying flexibility in how they function. As you think about what the word means, consider how people in your congregation would understand it.

> A *team* has a purpose while members of a *group* might have something in common yet no purpose.

Regardless of structure or size, purpose is the most important ingredient for teams. We need a clear reason for assembling a team. J. Richard Hackman names this as the first element for creating a "real work team" in his book, *Leading Teams: Setting the Stage for Great Performances*. He calls it a "team task" and uses the comparison of a string quartet.[8] A quartet needs to play together for the melody (purpose) to come across clearly and for the harmony to provide the richness. When it comes to health and wellness, finding that purpose can be a challenge since there

---

WHAT IS HEALTH MINISTRY?

Heath ministry is an organized effort at the congregational level to address health and wellness needs in the congregation or community. Health ministry takes many different forms. Take a close look at the books and articles referenced in the footnotes and appendices of this book. Go online to *Church Health Reader* and other websites dedicated to faith and health. Seek out your denomination or faith tradition's statement on faith and health.

WHO'S ON YOUR TEAM?

Start thinking early about who might be interested in being on a he[...]m (and whether they would want to be a part of it). Put out some feelers in informal conversations. How teams form varies from church to church. In some cases early conversations might include clergy, while in others you might want to build a strong case for a health team, including identifying team members, before you approach the leadership. Keep in mind what you know about how decisions turn into action in your setting.

are many topics to choose from. This is where a survey or assessment of your congregation could be most helpful.

Many of us, however, assemble a team because of a clear challenge that arises, such as visiting the sick, a need for a faith community nurse, the possibility of health coaching, or taking blood pressures. The strength of the team approach is that you will have multiple people (instruments) striving for the same purpose (melody), each with different tasks (harmonies) providing a rich or more complete health ministry. *mission statement?*

Although there is no single preferred model for a health team, it's safe to say there are several elements common to most. A health team:

- Consists of a small group of people from the congregation who meet regularly.
- Pursues a focus and purpose that meets a defined need.
- Knows the strengths of the congregation and understands what might motivate people in its congregation to meet this need.
- Addresses a need (or needs) using various methods such as education, support groups, pastoral care, health fairs, recreational activities, outreach, and referral.
- Maintains awareness of what is (or is not) happening in the congregation in terms of health and wellness, and possibly also the community at large.

This book presents a flexible structure for starting such a health team. It's up to you to shape it into a model that will work for you.

"TEAMING"

Some of the latest thinking in teamwork calls for us to think of team as a verb. Amy C. Edmonson, a professor at Harvard Business School, believes that when we face complex problems in our lives, we need to be able to respond quickly and flexibly. This response requires "teaming" in her view:

"Teaming is a verb. It is a dynamic activity, not a bounded, static entity. … Teaming is teamwork on the fly. It involves coordinating and collaborating without the benefit of stable team structures …"[9]

This sounds a lot like many of the challenges we face today in congregations. We need to work across lines to accomplish the large challenges we face. Such a framework might not be possible in all congregations, but it's worth thinking about how Edmonson's theory could aid the effectiveness of your health team.

RECOMMENDED READING
There are thousands of team and leadership books out there. If you want to dig into team theory, these volumes might be useful:

Teaming: How Organizations Learn, Innovate, and Compete in the Knowledge Economy by Amy C. Edmonson

Leading Teams: Setting the Stage for Great Performances by Richard Hackman

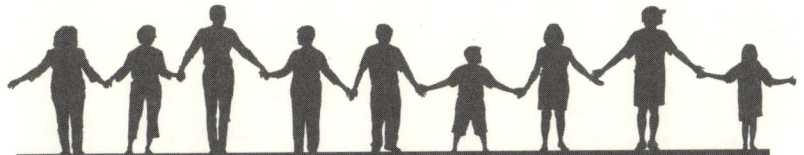

CHAPTER 1 SUMMARY

In this section, we looked at some foundational aspects of faith and health as well as some theories of teamwork. Remember that all of this takes time to develop. It might be a year before the team completes basic groundwork. If you are a person who wants to see immediate action, hang in there. Not all of the groundwork is introspective. During the process, you will raise the visibility of a health concern or wellness issue and educate your congregation about the pressing needs before us.

The Model of Jesus and His Disciples for Healing. Learn more about the Scriptural roots for your health ministry. Also, look into resources on health ministry. If your congregation belongs to a denomination, see if the denomination has a statement on faith and health.

Defining Health. Take a wholistic approach to health—one that takes into account people's attitudes, environments, and relationships.

Defining Team. A team is a group of people assembled for a clear purpose.

Jill's Story: A Feeling of Purpose

"There are a million ways to proclaim the good news, and we sell God short when we forget that, when we try to force ourselves into a narrow mold or fall silent because we cannot."
—Barbara Brown Taylor, author of *Gospel Medicine*[1]

A number of years ago, I went church shopping. I prayed my way through several denominations, various sizes of congregations, and traditional and contemporary worship styles. I listened closely to each word and nuance that might reveal a congregation's stance on theology and social justice. At each congregation I was acutely sensitive to how I was received. Did anyone other than the official greeters talk to me? Was I even noticed? Did it seem to make a difference that I was there?

Once being welcomed was a given, I wanted to move to the next level— being liked and valued. Would people care enough to discover my strengths, my gifts?

No matter what our situations, each of us has gifts. The more we use and develop these gifts, the richer our journey through life. A fortunate side effect of being valued and being asked to use our gifts is an increase in self-worth and often improved health. When others plug into our gifts, their lives become enriched and so do ours.

The church I chose was one week old on my first visit and very small, so the people were far more eager than most (dare I say desperate) to corral any talent that came along. Within weeks I was asked to teach adult education. That thrilled me. Later, I was asked to occasionally coordinate the food for donation and preparation for the homeless shelter. I dread recruiting people, but in the long run, it gave me satisfaction to accomplish something so worthwhile. I know I'm not alone in this feeling of purpose.

When you look at your community and congregation, what needs do you see? How do we build on the ministries we are already doing? What further ministries could grow from these well-founded motivations?

2
Finding Purpose:
What will your health team address?

"The healing ministry of congregations has often been limited to praying for and visiting the sick for the last few decades. There is nothing wrong with those activities, but there is much more that a church can do! And health ministry can be life-transforming for those who participate when the load is shared. This is a call to the body of Christ."
—Deborah Patterson, author of *The Healing Word: Preaching and Teaching Health Ministry*[1]

Once you've accomplished your general research into the foundational aspects of a health team, the next phase is determining what your health team will address. Think through these questions:

- What is your motivating force?
- What do you hope to achieve long term?
- What do you hope to achieve in the next six months? Over the next two years?

This phase will vary greatly depending on whether you already have a team that's working or if you are looking to create a team toward your chosen focus. It might also be better to engage your clergy from the very beginning. Remember to adjust each step to the specific context of your congregation.

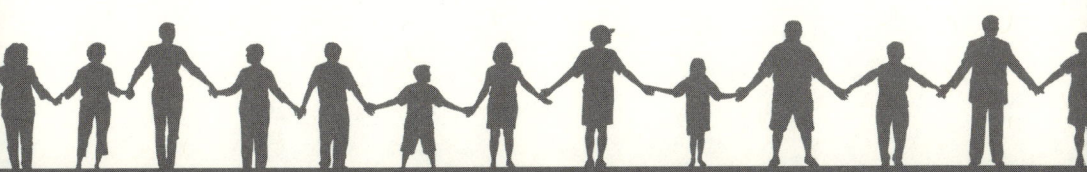

In this chapter, we will:
- **Walk** through a casual assessment of health ministry
- **Prepare** a health team purpose statement
- **Begin** conversations with leadership
- **Consider** congregational structure

A Casual Assessment

This first assessment will be casual in that you will not attempt to get the opinion of everyone in your congregation. Formal assessment comes later. (See Chapter 5.) Chances are you chose to create a health team because of certain needs that sparked your desire and so this initial assessment will be easy.

Health Team Purpose Statement

Your casual assessment will help you determine what the purpose of your team will be. It will also help you determine if your team will be short term or long term (depending how much you want to accomplish). But before you

---

QUESTIONS FOR CASUAL ASSESSMENT

As a team, determine what your congregation is currently doing that you believe promotes health. These questions will help you recognize what is happening.

- In what ways are various ministries promoting health?
- What health programs or projects are in place, such as small groups, a homeless shelter, hospital visitations, potlucks?
- What health expertise and experience exists among members?
- What health and wellness materials do you have such as books, pamphlets, videos, and liturgies?
- What health agencies does your town or city have and what services do they provide?
- What needs are not being met in your congregation or community? Write out a list, and then highlight three that you'd like to address.
- In what ways do you think your congregation could improve the ways it promotes wellness?
- What core strengths distinguish your congregation?
- What experience can you draw on? If other new ministries have been successful, talk with their leaders about what obstacles to watch for, how to navigate around them, or how to inspire people and leadership to be supportive.

---

go to the leadership to propose the formation of a health team, you will need a persuasive explanation. This will include:

- Why your congregation should be involved in health ministry. Define the link between faith and health.
- An acknowledgement of what your community is already doing.
- What you would like to accomplish with a health team and how this will benefit your congregation.

Because of the work done up to this point, you are ready to form a health team purpose statement. It should be concise while at the same time broad enough in scope to encompass everything the health team might do.

An example with a general purpose: *The health team shall foster the health ministry of our congregation.*

An example with a specific purpose: *The health team shall support people in need of food and shelter in our congregation and beyond.*

Go ahead. Give it a try. Don't strive for perfection because chances are you will alter it as you work through the phases of establishing a heath team, and it might change quite a bit after a discussion with clergy and congregational leadership.

Clergy and Staff Leadership

Your congregation's leadership is crucial to accomplishing your goals. This could vary depending on your denomination or tradition, yet most initiatives need the clergy's support. Discuss these four aspects initially with leadership:

- Why do you believe your congregation should be more involved in health? (This is where your research pays off.)
- How might a health team affect the congregation?
- What will be leadership's role with the health team?
- How might a health team fit—or not fit—into the organizational structure?

Note, I used the word *discuss*. While part of this meeting with leadership involves selling your idea, you also need to listen to their comments. Incorporate their perspectives into your plan. Make it clear that you value their experience and insights.

- How do leaders understand your focus or purpose?
- Has the congregation addressed a health team in the past?
- How might a health team affect the congregation?
- Are leaders in favor of establishing a health team?
- What will their role be with a health team?
- How would a health team fit into the organizational structure?

Also, take a look at your clergy's leadership style. Do they tend to set a strong direction and let the congregation run with the project or work? Do they want to be involved in each step along the way? How strong is the leadership vision? How present is leadership in the actual day-to-day operations? These questions will help you consider how much you need to include leadership in the early decision-making process or whether you simply need the blessing of the leadership to let you begin the work. Either way (and the variations in between) can work for the project.

Incorporate church leadership's perspectives into your plan. Make it clear that your value their insight.

Bringing out any assumptions from the beginning is a good practice, so you aren't surprised by leadership's response down the road. What is *their* understanding of your purpose? Is this something that the congregation has tried to address in the past? Are they in favor of establishing a health team?

After meeting with the leadership, write down what you learned. It's useful at this point to assess whether you need to adjust your direction or proposed purpose and meet with leadership again.

Congregational Structure

Your congregation's structure, such as committees and other governing bodies, will determine how your health team operates. At this point, it is helpful to verify what steps are required to start a new initiative in your congregation. This will vary for each community depending on your denomination or tradition. For some, it depends on how long this team will work together. Will it be long-term or only short-term for a given project? Will you need to work through an existing committee or will yours be a group that stands alone?

Soon you will be talking with your congregation about your intentions and asking for their suggestions. Think through how best to do that in your circumstances. If you involve people early, they are more likely to support the work. A few of them might ask to join your team.

CULTURE AND CONGREGATIONS

How will your congregation best understand the need to create a health team? Here are some possible responses:

- a critical neighborhood need
- a pressing issue within the congregation
- a biblical mandate
- a social justice issue
- a pastoral care issue

Consider the culture or tradition and people of your congregation. Discuss with your working team and leadership the most effective way to present your focus to them.

ADDRESSING HEALTH DISPARITIES AND POVERTY

If you have decided to address a health disparity or a poverty-related issue in your community, it's important to explore the various aspects of your chosen issue. In particular, a lack of hope and purpose can impact a person's health. One study, which followed a group of disenfranchised people, found that "35 percent of the suffering could not be accounted for." They concluded it was people's lack of hope. The people "had no faith that they themselves could change their own destiny, that their decisions would make a difference in their lives."[2]

Unnatural Causes: Is Inequality Making Us Sick? is a must-see documentary series for anyone looking to take on health disparities in their community. The series, broadcast on the Public Broadcasting Service, examines how socioeconomic and racial inequality affect health. It includes seven episodes, with the first episode, "In Sickness and in Wealth," introducing the main themes of the series. The website features additional resources such as a primer on health inequality: www.unnaturalcauses.org

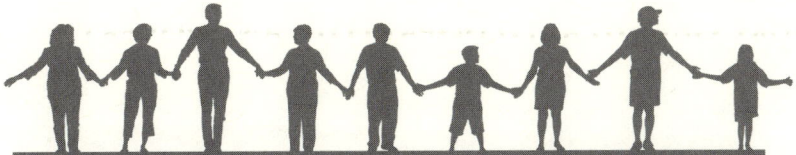

CHAPTER 2 SUMMARY

You are on your way! You and the other members of your team have pooled your thoughts about what is already happening in your congregation in terms of health. You have also listed some of the needs of your community. By no means are these lists complete, but they give you a rough idea of where you might be headed. You have also written a basic health team purpose statement based on these findings.

You understand that for a health team to succeed, leadership support is crucial. You have talked with the leaders (staff and non-staff) of your congregation. Based on your discussion, you have written up an account of that meeting and considered whether you might need to adjust how or what you hope to accomplish.

A Casual Assessment. This assessment quickly determines—to the best of your knowledge or your team's collective knowledge —what your congregation is currently doing to promote health. A more systematic approach for a formal assessment occurs later.

Health Team Purpose Statement. Try writing a basic health team purpose statement. See if you can relate it to the congregation's overall mission.

Clergy and Staff Leadership. For a health team to succeed, the leadership support is crucial. Talk with the leaders (staff and non-staff) of your congregation.

Congregational Structure. Your congregation's structure, such as committees and other governing bodies, will determine how your health team operates. Discover what steps are required to start a new initiative in your congregation.

Henry's Story

"When we help, we see others as weak. When we fix them, we see them as broken. When we serve, we see others as holy."
—Rev. Henry Fischer[1]

When Rev. Henry Fischer went to Germany to work in a group home, he lived with eight men who were developmentally delayed. He was told that that label wasn't possible in German. Instead the people were considered "relationally advanced." Pastor Fischer thought he was going to Germany to help these people, but instead they showed him how to love:

> I no sooner approached the front door than Wolfgang came out of nowhere and hugged me. Pinning my arms against my sides ... he said, "Brother Fischer, Jesus told me that I was supposed to teach you and show you how to love." And he and others like him did. But it took time. All I am today I owe to Wolfgang and the others in Bethel who acted as Jesus Christ's Secret Agents who led me to a deeper understanding of myself, finding a fuller humanity and moving on to wholeness. Discovering that in ministry, Jesus Christ meets us coming and going. There is no giving or receiving. There is just being.[2]

Rev. Fischer, a retired Lutheran minister, demonstrates that words are powerful, to the point of altering our attitudes and perceptions. Donning the mentality of service, we, the servers, usually end up gaining the most. In our health ministries we need to move beyond the mentality that we are there to "help" others. Instead we need to recognize that we are there to "serve."

In the elementary school where I work, children with a myriad of disabilities are included in regular classrooms as much as possible. Sometimes I wonder how much they benefit, especially in the upper grades. I rarely wonder, though, about the benefits to the rest of the class. The children are learning to be comfortable with people who used to be locked away in institutions— people who scared me when I was in grade school. Children at River Woods Elementary push their friends in wheelchairs and play soccer with friends who have Down syndrome. These children who work in partnership with children with disabilities develop strategies for learning and teaching as well as patience. They experience joy when their friend breaks out in a smile because he finally understood the math. They are proud for the girl with autism when she presents an oral report.

An initial phase of serving is welcoming. Whether we want to serve within or beyond our congregations, people must feel welcome. This goes beyond having a wheelchair ramp or greeters at the door. Once people are in your building will others continue to talk with them? Will they be invited into a circle of conversation at the coffee hour or will they have to initiate the conversation? Will the people sitting next to them make an effort to find out who they are beyond just their name?

This sort of welcoming moves beyond acknowledging someone's presence to valuing the person. How can we serve in a way that allows us to discover and receive the gifts people have? What needs to be changed so that congregations issue a genuine invitation to participate? How do we welcome people into our health teams and also into our project or activities?

3
Assemble the Team
Who will work alongside you?

"If you light a lamp for someone, it will brighten your own path."
—The Buddha

Everyone wants to be valued—to have others look at them and see their gifts. This can be difficult, especially when someone has an obvious disability as in the Henry Fischer story. There are situations in our congregations where we're ready to "help those people," but we forget about "serving." When we are deciding what needs to address, it's tempting to want to reach out to people whom we regard as needy. We want our building to be wheelchair accessible; we want to provide shelter for the homeless and information on preventing illness. While these are worthy aims, the effects will be longer lasting if we first acknowledge the strengths of people and utilize their gifts.

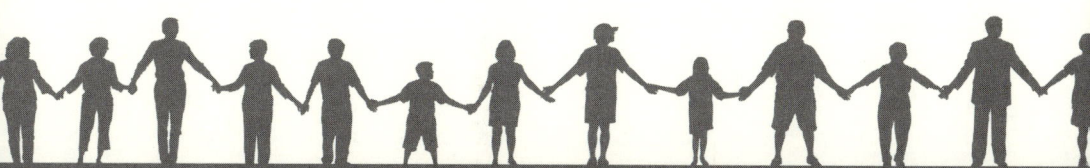

In this chapter, we will:

- **Explore** giftedness within the team
- **Increase** awareness of congregational strengths and weaknesses
- **Discover** like-mindedness beyond the congregation

Valuing the Health Team

Your team will consist of people in the congregation interested in promoting the health focus. A balance of health professionals and non-health professionals is ideal, with team members who represent all demographics in your congregation. The non-health professionals can help the health professionals understand the perspective of most of the people in the community. They also might be the ones who have the talent for organizing, making contact with other organizations, finding funding, and other key roles. Include people who understand the inner workings of your congregation—how things get done in your particular setting.

"How then does a congregation have the strength to pour itself out for the community? Like most living phenomena, it is almost impossibly complex to engineer. Fortunately, this is an organic process to be nurtured, not a machine to be engineered. Think like a gardener, and it becomes easier to see."[1]

—Gary Gunderson, author of Deeply Woven Roots

Learn about the talents and skills of each member of the health team. Begin by having people involved in the health team share what they believe they do well and how their abilities might be an asset to the team. Welcome conversation about a wide spectrum of gifts—health practices, organizing abilities, carpentry skills, planning, networking with people and other health organizations—and talk about how each gift might contribute to your efforts. Some individuals may already be involved in health ministry in some way, whether in the church or in the community. Would they like to continue it and make it stronger?

Next talk about those aspects of your current health ministry that are not as strong (all the while being sensitive to anyone who has taken part in them). Should these activities continue as part of the new team's work? Are the gifts of the new team the right abilities to strengthen something that is weak?

Finally move on to brainstorming new ideas. Knowing your strengths and weaknesses, what can you realistically do? What is missing? Do you need to seek out more team members to bring needed strengths?

Valuing the Congregation

Once you have a good idea of your team members' talents and skills, you will want to examine your congregation's strengths. Ask your team to talk about the strengths of individuals in your congregation. What does your congregation do well that promotes health and wellness? For instance, are members taking meals to shut-ins? Is there an exercise group? A new health team will not take over these ministries, but you will want to talk to the people involved and find out how you might support what they're doing.

Apart from current health ministries, evaluate these dimensions of congregational life:

- How does the congregation handle conflict?
- How do members deal with change?
- In what ways are visitors welcomed?
- How do you accommodate people with special needs, whether physical, developmental, or emotional?
- Who has strength in a time of crisis? Who is likely to offer assistance?

You will accomplish your goals much sooner and the effects will last longer if you utilize your gifts. When you have an idea of your community's gifts you are in a better position to address some of the needs by leveraging strengths.

Once you have an overall idea of the strengths within your team and congregation, take some time to assess your purpose. Revisit your purpose statement. Does it still fit? Do you need to alter it? Who will best help achieve that purpose? Are these people already on your team or are there others you would like to recruit? For instance, if you are looking to begin a specific wellness initiative, such as a garden or an exercise course, how can you find out who has those skills?

Partnerships in the Wider Community

It's important to look beyond your congregation's walls for potential partners and to assure that you are not duplicating work already being done. Part of your early research was to become more aware of agencies in your town and the services they offer. At this point in developing your health team, it's helpful to talk with people from other congregations and health agencies to learn from their experiences. You may be beginning a new health team in your congregation, but this does not mean you cannot benefit from those who have gone before you in similar work. If there are overlapping interests, see how you can work together. Partnerships can be key to this work.

CASE STUDY: HABITAT FOR HUMANITY

People tend to thrive when we put their gifts to work. Think about Habitat for Humanity. The houses they build are not given away. The future owners provide hundreds of hours of sweat equity, and over the years they repay their no-interest loans. Helping to build and buy their own houses gives people a sense of pride, accomplishment and appreciation. It teaches practical skills that can be used in the future.

CHAPTER 3 SUMMARY

It's time to assemble the team or think about who to add to your team. Find the gifts in your congregation. Value each individual. Value what each ministry already does well. Learn from them and receive their gifts. Your initiatives and projects will thrive if you nurture people's gifts.

Valuing the Health Team. Your team will do a self-assessment of their gifts and talents.

Valuing the Congregation. As a team, you will do a similar assessment of your congregation. Determine what the congregation does well. That will inform you about how to move forward with a specific health ministry.

Partnerships in the Wider Community. Once you have finished these assessments it's time to begin thinking about partnerships with the wider community. What resources are out there? How will you be able to plug into them?

Jesse's Story

"If people are hurting and rejected, they don't care what the Bible says. What they want is relief from the pain."[1]
—Jesse Stinson, founder of The Sharing Group

When Jesse Stinson's life fractured in 1964, this straightforward truth shone the light of healing. Overnight he went from having a job and a family to being in a hospital that treated severe mental illness. For ten months he moved through the process of first admitting that he was sick and then understanding his illness. While in treatment, he discovered that talking to others helped him find healing.

When he was released from the hospital, with multiple mental health diagnoses, Jesse faced the challenge of putting his life back together. Because he had benefited from being part of a support group while hospitalized, he began "The Sharing Group" in a Birmingham, Alabama church. Since 1964, thousands of people with a range of mental illnesses have passed through The Sharing Group. The group has welcomed homeless individuals as well as people in stable employment with illnesses ranging from depression to schizophrenia.

Jesse Stinston's vision was to help people in the church welcome those with mental illness and to help those who were ill realize that the church does not have to be one more place where they feel rejection or don't know how to fit in. The Sharing Group has been a ministry of healing that addresses an area of illness many churches are uncomfortable with.

The Sharing Group is organized around three simple principles. First, share with others. Everyone comes with a story, and the group is a safe place to tell it. Second, find support to heal. The group gives people a place to feel accepted while seeking healing in body and spirit. Third, gather strength to go on. Many members have gotten better, secured jobs, found stable housing, reconciled with family, or gone to college.

A church can make a valuable contribution to a focused health ministry like The Sharing Group by providing meeting space and something as simple as meals or refreshments that encourage people to attend—and thus take a first step toward being less isolated in their illness.

4
Listening to the Congregation:
What is the most effective approach?

"We should listen with the ears of God …"
—Dietrich Bonhoeffer[1]

You have your purpose. You are building your team, and learning about the gifts and talents of the congregation. It's time to dig deeper into the specific needs and assets of your congregation and the larger community. You will discover even more along your way. Be sure to keep your focus, though. It can be overwhelming to look at all the information that conversation or a more formal assessment gives back to you.

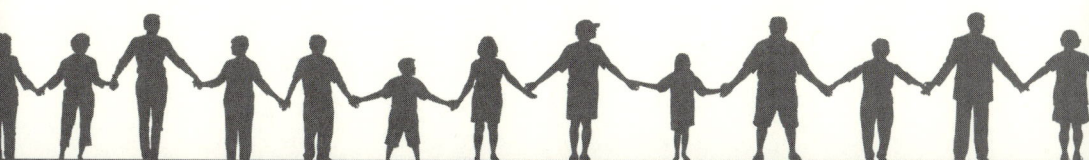

In this chapter, we will:

- **Understand** assessment fundamentals
- **Review** options for methods of assessment
- **Envision** conversations beyond the congregation

Assessment Fundamentals

There are several formal and informal ways to assess the congregation, including anonymous written surveys, multiple choice questions, open-ended questions, personal interviews, and meeting with other ministry groups for discussion of key questions. Whether you use written or spoken formats, listening well is the most important skill to employ during this step. To be an active listener means opening yourself up to hear the needs, dreams, and frustrations of each person. Such listening will strengthen your purpose and resolve! Because the newly formed team has been discussing important questions already, be sure to ask for information and input that does not steer responses toward a particular conclusion. This is the phase for taking the conversation outside of your team and hearing perspectives you might not have thought of before. Going beyond the health team for input will make your assessment more comprehensive. By seeking out the opinions of your entire congregation you will get a more accurate reading and you will also give many people ownership in the project.

Ideally an assessment would include three main outcomes:

1. Identify the talents and skills present in your congregation. You began this work in Chapter 3, but it is an ongoing process as your project evolves.
2. Recognize the health and wellness activities currently happening within your walls and beyond that might support or overlap with your purpose. By widening the discussion, you may discover there is more going on than you realized.
3. Discover your congregation's or larger community's current state of health and wellness and how that relates to your purpose and goals. Assessment results will confirm the path you are on or help you more clearly define what you want to do going forward.

LISTENING

To truly listen to others, give them your full attention—without multi-tasking. Be receptive and open to what they say, even if you don't agree. Make eye contact and show by your posture that you are listening. Ask questions for clarification, but don't give advice or your opinion. Be patient.

Dietrich Bonhoeffer was a German theologian who vocally opposed the Nazi regime. In his writing, he says, "There is also a kind of listening with half an ear that presumes already to know what the other person has to say. This impatient, inattentive listening really despises the other Christian and finally is only waiting to get a chance to speak and thus to get rid of the other. This sort of listening is no fulfillment of our task. And it is certain that here, too, in our attitude toward other Christians we simply see reflected our own relationship to God. ... Christians have forgotten that the ministry of listening has been entrusted to them by the one who is indeed the great listener and in whose work they are to participate. We should listen with the ears of God, so that we can speak the Word of God." [2]

You have gained some of this information through informal methods and conversation. In a formal assessment, the goal is to reduce the guesswork by gathering information in a manner that will allow you to identify trends and patterns in the responses to your questions. In the course of your assessment, regardless of the type you settle on, frame questions in a way that does not assume a base of knowledge about health or health ministry. You will want to be able to use the information you gather to answer these questions.

- What do people in our congregation perceive we are already doing for health and wellness?
- In what ways are people in your congregation caring for others?
- In what ways do people in our congregation see faith and health connecting?
- What are the health-related needs and desires of individuals and the congregation as a whole?
- Is the congregation more interested in addressing health needs within the congregation or in a health-related form of outreach?

Methods of Assessment

There is no one perfect way to gather information. You might find a combination of methods reaches the most people.

Written survey. A formal survey, either paper or electronic, might be an effective way to reach the most people in your congregation. You will want to customize the survey to meet your specific project or aim. You can administer the survey during a regular meeting time of your congregation, such as weekly worship, or take it to meetings of groups that meet throughout the week. It may be worthwhile to seek out the technological expertise to make a survey available online so people can complete it at their leisure. You do all of these things in order to reach the most people possible.

Your health ministry does not have to be an island, but rather part of the health and wellness landscape of your community.

Academic survey. If your congregation is large, you might want to partner with a local college or hospital that has knowledge of how to conduct larger-scale surveys. Academics, in particular, are delighted to share their expertise to address a health and wellness need!

Small group conversations. Visit with people in their homes, during coffee hour, and any other opportune time. Ask for a few minutes during committee meetings or choir practice. Make sure you reach into all the demographics of your congregation, including the youth. Listen to stories. Use a prepared prompt of questions so that you ask everybody the same thing. Is there particular interest in exercise? Nutrition? Heart health? Stress management?

Hopefully during this time of listening you will not only learn about the state of health and wellness in your congregation, but you will also find more people who want to participate. They might not want to sign up for the health team, but they might be willing to help out occasionally with a given project.

Town hall-style meetings. A town hall-style meeting will not be the best format for gathering individual information about health concerns, but it may be an effective way to introduce the vision of a health team and encourage engagement in the conversation about health and wellness in your congregation. Plan an agenda that will allow you to make a brief presentation of key questions and then invite questions and discussion. No decisions will be made in this meeting. It is simply a method of gathering input from a larger group.

Clergy conversations. Another effective way to assess the health needs is to talk with all the staff members and with the committees or groups in your congregation. Because of their work they will know of some unmet needs. Chances are they will have ideas how some of these needs can be met. Also, remember that every one of these people is probably doing some form of health ministry. (Just the act of meeting monthly and coming to know each other through the work you do promotes health.) Acknowledge that! Find out how your team might be supportive.

Beyond the Walls of Your Congregation

Reaching into the community can be more complicated, but if you plan to do outreach, it is necessary. Start by talking with other congregations and health care agencies.

- What are they already doing?
- What do they wish could be done?
- Has a health needs assessment already been done?
- What current projects could your congregation tap into?
- What could you do together?
- Is there a speakers forum?

Remember, your health ministry does not have to be an island, but rather part of the health and wellness landscape of your community or denomination.

SURVEY IDEAS

If you decide that a survey during worship one week will reach the most people, find ways to incorporate a health theme into the service. Here are a few ideas:

- Ask the minister to preach about health.

- Have a representative from the health team describe her or his dreams for the health of the congregation.

- Use prayers or hymns that resonate with your health focus.

- Tuck survey sheets into the bulletin. People can fill them out during the service, then return them as part of their offering.

- Since not everyone will be at the service, have options such as a survey in the weekly or monthly newsletter or at events throughout the week.

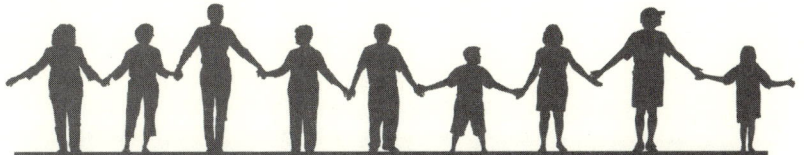

CHAPTER 4 SUMMARY

A formal assessment phase takes the conversation about health and wellness wider than the experiences or impressions of the health team. Establish goals for your assessment process and plan your tools to help you answer key questions.

Assessment Fundamentals. In a formal assessment, the goal is to reduce the guesswork by gathering information in a manner that will allow you to identify trends and patterns in the responses to your questions. In the course of your assessment, regardless of the type you settle on, frame questions in a way that does not assume a base of knowledge about health or health ministry. Look at the questions your team has been considering from the perspective of the congregation.

Methods of Assessment. Methods may include written surveys, on paper or electronically, academic assistance with a large survey project, small group conversations, a town hall-style meeting, and clergy conversations. No matter which form of assessment you choose, listening is key. It takes practice to open up our minds and ears to all people in your congregation.

Beyond the Walls of Your Congregation. Eventually you will have conversations beyond the walls of your congregation. Continue to be receptive to the thoughts of individuals involved in health ministry in your community. Dream about how you can partner with them.

Cindi's Story

"Tell me, what is it you plan to do with your one wild and precious life?"
—Mary Oliver in her poem "The Summer Day"

Mary Oliver's poem implores us to take the time we have on this earth and to make the most of it. This challenge is even greater when we face serious illness or permanent disabilities. People have done it, often through the support of their congregation and its partnerships with the wider community. But it means taking risks and stepping on out with faith. It often requires building partnerships across the congregation and into the community.

A close friend of mine has a son with Down syndrome. When Adam was born, Cindi and her husband, Art, were devastated. This was not supposed to happen—it wasn't in the plan.

Cindi spent the first months of Adam's life caring for him and his older brother. She and Adam participated in an early intervention program, giving Adam every opportunity for progress and Cindi a network of supportive friends and professionals. She did it all, through a fog of depression. She was angry at God and she was angry at her church for offering no outreach—no visits from a pastoral caller, not even a chicken dinner.

When Adam was about five months old, Cindi took him to the pediatrician who proceeded to list everything that could go wrong with Adam. That was the last thing Cindi needed. She couldn't hold back her tears. A doctor with an ounce of sensitivity would have put her arm around Cindi. This doctor yelled at Cindi, admonishing her to be strong for her husband.

At six months, Adam got sick. Cindi's friends in the early intervention program recommended a new doctor. Bracing herself, Cindi took Adam in. The doctor examined Adam, showing respect for him throughout the process. She commented on his great muscle tone. "Keep doing whatever you're doing," she said. This was Cindi's first outside affirmation and it was the turning point for her healing.

It was several more months before Cindi made it through the grief process. Adam was at least a year old before hope was steady in her life. Although grieving is difficult business, having done it she was able to move forward a little stronger and definitely wiser. Many parents of children with disabilities never resolve their grief and so those feelings remain major barriers to them.

Over the next several years Cindi continued to work with Adam at home and through the early intervention and early childhood programs. She became very pragmatic and realistic. She learned to strategize for Adam's future, trying to keep at least three years ahead. Having done a lot of research, she and Art had chosen the route they felt would be best for Adam. They set out to make changes in the schools, their church, the city, and even the state.

Then when Adam was ten, Cindi was diagnosed with Leber's Hereditary Optic Neuropathy. She was going blind. She now had three sons to care for and she worked as a journalist. How would she manage? But she was determined, believing she had to set a positive example for her sons who might one day develop this condition.

Adam became her inspiration. His persistence to learn inspired her. "In learning to tie his shoes, to zip his jacket, to talk, he tried and tried. He never gave up," said Cindi, "so how could I give up?"

The suffering Cindi went through made her stronger, more passionate, more courageous and more pragmatic. She developed an eye for seeing everyone as a reflection of God. She's had the privilege of meeting people who've been thrown away—considered hopeless—and she has watched them succeed.

After losing her vision, Cindi returned to school and earned her masters in social work. She worked at a Catholic parish, followed by a Lutheran church as a coordinator for ministry to people with disabilities. Cindi finds ways to include (not just welcome) people into the life of the church. She and a friend founded Pathfinders Consulting Service. They work with parents and professionals, helping them create caring communities for their people with disabilities.

Cindi and Art, along with two other families, started a co-op. They bought a greenhouse, which serves as a job training site for adults with disabilities. Fifty-five families (all who have a family member with a disability) bought into it. Such work demonstrates that we are truly stronger together. Further, this story shows the crucial role that congregations have to play in building these partnerships and teams for health ministry.

Through Cindi, and others like her, I receive energy and hope.

Congregations need to be places where people—whether they have a disability or not—take risks. When we take risks, growth occurs. I love the saying that "churches should comfort the afflicted and afflict the comfortable." Ideally, when we are in pain, our congregation is there, walking with us every step. It challenges our thinking and prods us to action. Only by taking risks, however small, will we bring about significant changes to ourselves and others. Our congregation can encourage us to take those risks, and we can help to make God's nature come to fruition in the world.

Our lives will not be easy or always accepted by others as the "right" way. We might rock the boat. We might not fit in, but we will have creative, transforming lives. Jesus did not remove himself from his own suffering or that of others. Jesus welcomed the sick and the disenfranchised. His ministry lifted people up.

5
Formalizing Your Team:
What are your goals and objectives?

As he walked by the Sea of Galilee, he saw two brothers, Simon, who is called Peter, and Andrew his brother, casting a net into the sea—for they were fishermen. And he said to them, "Follow me, and I will make you fish for people." Immediately they left their nets and followed him. As he went from there, he saw two other brothers, James son of Zebedee and his brother John, in the boat with their father Zebedee, mending their nets, and he called them. Immediately they left the boat and their father, and followed him.
—Matthew 4:18–22

It's time to step out. You are ready to formalize the team and present yourselves and your purpose to the community. You have honed this purpose with the team. You have educated your congregation and you have sought their advice. You have identified one or more needs that are not being met. All of this information will help you shape your goals and objectives.

Some structure is needed (even in the most unstructured setting) if the team is to survive. It might be a board, a committee of another board, or simply a group of people who meet regularly, but only for one year. The structure depends on your purpose, your context and your goals.

You will want to hold a team meeting and have each team member discuss the following aspects outlined in this step, in particular their time commitment.

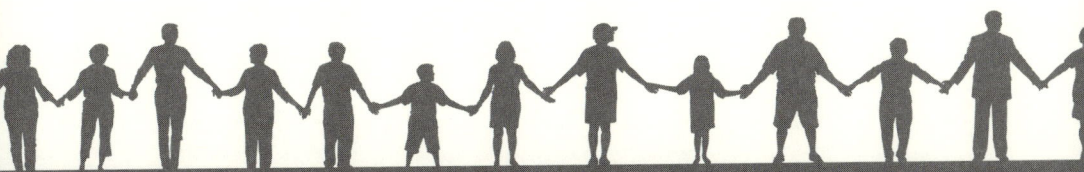

In this chapter, we will:
- **Assign** responsibilities for how the health team will function
- **Plan** communication with leaders and other agencies
- **Make** a budget
- **Set out** specific tasks to accomplish

Time Commitment and Formal Roles

Members should commit themselves for a given time period and regularly attend meetings. (Meetings also should be open to non-members except when a discussion requires confidentiality.) Some discussion can be done online or with conference calls, but there is no substitute for being together and strengthening your relationships.

Formal roles might include the following:

- *Coordinator.* The coordinator is responsible for the overall ministry of the health team. This person provides direction, sets the agenda, and supports members of the team. While the coordinator oversees all projects, he or she is not in charge of all of them. The coordinator reports to the congregation's leadership and facilitates dialogue between the team and the rest of the congregation. The coordinator fosters a caring atmosphere among the team members. This might mean taking a few minutes to let people share about their personal lives or provide a simple devotion. When people feel cared for, they will be able to do a better job caring for others.

The beauty of the health team is that so much can be done at little or no cost.

- *Secretary.* The secretary is responsible for keeping a record of all that occurs. He or she will take notes on the meetings and send copies to all the team members. Other team members can send notes to the secretary regarding projects they are working on to then be emailed to the rest of the team.

- *Communications.* If there are enough people on your team, consider a communications person. Otherwise this role probably will fall to the coordinator. This person makes sure that blurbs appear in your congregation's newsletters or perhaps get published in local newspapers—whatever you can think of to let as many people as possible know what you are doing.

- *Current Staff or Special Hires.* If your congregation has a faith community nurse, ideally this person is a member of the team and therefore participates in the same way a member does. As a member of the staff, he or she is the liaison between the health team and the rest of the staff. From talking with nurses I've learned that it usually works best if the nurse is not the coordinator. The nurse's time can be more wisely spent providing trained care to others.

Each project might also require adding people to your staff (on a short-term or long-term basis) to accomplish specific tasks. This will become clearer when you outline the goals and objectives (later in this chapter). There are logistics here to consider such as your congregation's policies around contracting with outside vendors or individuals.

- *Team members.* Members of the health team support the coordinator and each other. The coordinator provides the direction but does not make all of the decisions. The entire committee discusses ideas or issues and makes decisions. The team organizes and carries out specific projects. Team members act as a catalyst to groups within the congregation.

Communication with Leadership and Governance

What will be the means of communication between the health team and the staff or other groups in the congregation? Through communication the health team can continually learn what others are doing and what others would like to see happen. It might be appropriate to work through an existing group. For example, you might ask the education team if you can do a session on faith and health for either adults or children.

You can also encourage other groups or individuals to promote health. Existing teams or new teams might take on health initiatives such as blood drives or crisis intervention. Cheer them on! Ask how you can be of assistance. Make sure someone on your team serves as a liaison.

With regular communication, your health team will not overstep its boundaries and it will have a greater impact. When contact is frequent, staff and other groups will have a greater tendency to remember the health aspects of their ministries.

Communication with People and Agencies Beyond Your Congregation

Networking can multiply your effectiveness. Boost your own numbers at courses or programs by inviting the community. And take advantage of what the community offers. For instance, why offer a grief workshop when the local hospital is running one? Bring in speakers from local agencies. Ask the local hospital to file the advanced directives of your members. Be aware of community resources so you can refer your members to them. By developing relationships with other health agencies you will learn of offerings you didn't know existed. This will benefit your members. When they come to you asking for help, you will know how and where to access the services they need.

Budget

It's finally time to discuss budget. Until now there's been no mention of money because it's important to let your team dream and explore possibilities without hindering the discussion with budgetary restraints. The beauty of the health team is that so much can be done at little or no cost. You probably have many people resources within your congregation. Local hospitals and health agencies will often supply speakers, training and materials at no cost. Ministry such as visiting people who are sick, working to include people with special needs and leading support groups cost only your time. Yet you must eventually consider your financial resources, and as you shape your specific goals and objectives, it is wise to start sketching out some budget items. A specific line item budget for your first year will wait until after you have settled on your goals and objectives in Step 5.

> There is no substitute for being together and strengthening your relationships.

Tasks, Goals, and Objectives

You probably are brimming, if not overwhelmed, with ideas regarding what the health team's goals and objectives might be, but take care to be realistic. Your team's resources and energy are limited. Depending on the complexity of your purpose, you might start with just one goal or attempt three. Just remember, it's better to start small. It's much easier to add goals than to take them away.

In developing your objectives, be specific. If your goal is to improve the mental health of your congregation, your objectives might be to start a resource library and have a panel discussion on stress management. If you are working with a local mental health agency you might offer space in your building for a support group.

While you are planning your goals and objectives, keep in mind:

- the learning from your assessment
- available resources, needs of the congregation and surrounding area
- how ideas succeed in your congregation
- what the obstacles are and how you will deal with them
- how you can network with other congregations and health agencies

If it is appropriate, make a convincing presentation to the leadership or the entire congregation. Once you have gotten their go-ahead, keep them informed of your progress so they will continue to be supportive.

From Cindi's story, we know that she faced great adversity in her life, yet she found a way to build a vital ministry within her community. You are in the midst of such risk-taking. Be sure not to lose that purpose that Jesus modeled for us in his ministry. Cross unexpected lines. Face obstacles with love and forgiveness. Support each other along the way.

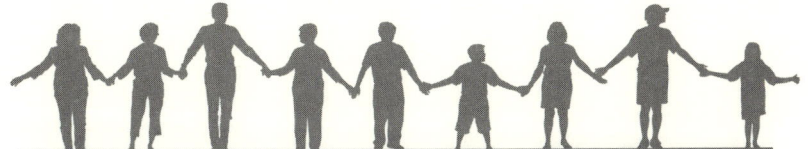

CHAPTER 5 SUMMARY

At the end of this chapter, the following structural items will need to be agreed upon: meeting time and place, approximate number of people on the team, formal roles, expectation of time commitment, to whom the team is accountable, and the budget.

Formal Roles. You might have already determined who does what along the way. If so, great. As staid as these roles might sound you need to know you is responsible for what. Someone needs to provide direction and pull findings together into a usable form. Someone needs to keep a record of meetings and all the findings. And don't forget that key to the success of your team is communication.

Communication with Leadership and Governance. With regular communication, your health team will not overstep its boundaries and it will have a greater impact. When contact is frequent, staff and other groups will have a greater tendency to remember the health aspects of their ministries.

Communication with People and Agencies Beyond Your Congregation. By developing relationships with other health agencies you will learn of offerings you didn't know existed. This will benefit your members. When they come to you asking for help, you will know how and where to access the services they need.

Budget. Until now there's been no mention of money because it's important to let your team dream and explore possibilities without hindering the discussion with budgetary restraints. The beauty of the health team is that so much can be done at little or no cost.

Tasks, Goals, and Objectives. Your team's resources and energy are limited. Depending on the complexity of your purpose, you might start with just one goal or attempt three. It's better to start small. It's much easier to add goals than to take them away.

Alex's Story

Dory: Hey there, Mr. Grumpy Gills. When life gets you down,
do you wanna know what you've gotta do?
Marlin: No I don't wanna know.
Dory: [singing] Just keep swimming. Just keep swimming.
—*Finding Nemo*, Pixar Animation Studies, 2003

It was after the birth of his second child was born that Alex began to really feel stressed. And then he felt guilty for feeling so stressed. He was a young successful doctor with a loving wife and two wonderful children. He had settled in a city he enjoyed and established a medical practice that enabled him to work with grateful people on interesting issues, and to teach medical school students at the beginning of their careers. Yet Alex was burned out. Moreover, he saw even greater burnout happening all around him. The medical students he worked with, barely a few years into their studies, were already beginning to question why they had endeavored to try medical school in the first place. All around him, Alex felt the frustration of the health care system weighing in on him, his family and his friends.

Luckily, Alex had a community to turn to at his church. He voiced his frustrations with other health care professionals and came up with a plan. Once a week, he invited students to a class or discussion with other medical professionals. They openly discussed working with challenging patients, available community resources, new models for how to provide health care, and even how to maintain an active prayer life in the hospital system. Through the discussions, Alex and his students were able to reconnect with what inspired them to the medical profession in the first place—the chance to help people who needed it. He felt reenergized for his profession, and reconnected with his students.

Health ministry is not always a short endeavor or an easy calling. We have to find ways to encourage ourselves and our team, reconnecting with our passions and avoiding the ever-present temptation for fatigue and burnout. Alex shows us how important it is to have a community to help. Making sure your health ministry team is supportive of each other is key to maintaining your goals, celebrating successes, and continuing to grow.

6
And Action!
What is your plan for the future?

"How far that little candle throws his beams!
So shines a good deed in a weary world."
—*The Merchant of Venice* by William Shakespeare

Now it's time to develop a plan of action for the first year. Brainstorm what you would ideally like to accomplish. From that list choose a few goals that are possible to accomplish. Be realistic. (Keep the rest of the ideas for the future.) Identify one person who will be in charge of carrying out each goal and who will be accountable to the health team coordinator. Set some target dates. The objectives under each goal will be decided by the person(s) responsible for it.

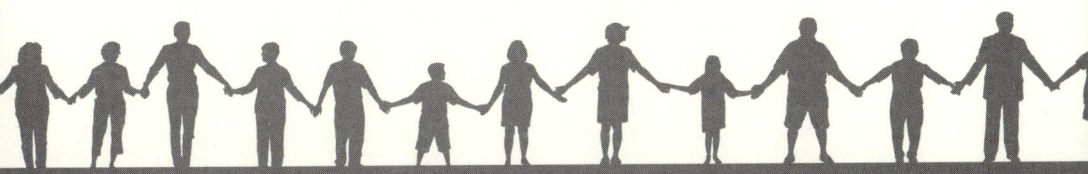

In this chapter, we will:
- **Recognize** the importance of visibility and communication
- **Avoid** burnout

Visibility and Communication with the Congregation

From the beginning you've involved your congregation. You've begun to educate them about your vision for the health team, and you have invited their input. Keep up that visibility. Not only do you want your congregation to know who you are and what you're doing, you want them to "own" the health team and be proud of its work.

Here are some ideas to keep this visibility alive:

- Include an item about the health team in the newsletter and the bulletin.
- Update people on the progress of the health team during the announcements at worship.
- Thank people for their participation in the assessment survey and let them know what you plan to do as a result of their input.
- Schedule an event like a potluck that will attract people to spend an evening discussing faith and health. At this event reiterate the links between faith and health and why your congregation should strengthen its health ministry. Present the health team concept and all that you see it entailing. Include a more detailed summary of what you learned from the assessment. Share some of your dreams for the team. Set aside a large block of time for questions, suggestions and discussion. Ask for volunteers who would be interested in serving on the team or helping out in other ways (no commitment necessary as of yet). Let people know the time and place of the next health team meeting. Encourage them to come, even if they don't want to be a member. After the event, follow up with the people who showed interest. Find out specifically in what capacity and in what areas they would like to serve.

Note on Burnout

When you're contemplating a health team or new forms of health ministry, burnout doesn't seem to be anywhere on the horizon. At this stage the ideas are energizing. But just ask any health care professional—burnout is real.

People who are busy caring for others often forget to care for themselves. And while it may seem selfish to care for ourselves, the healthier we are, the more we are able to care for others. With that in mind, here are some thoughts on avoiding burnout.

Make sure you have the support of your congregation and its leaders. Without their support, you are limited in what you can accomplish. With their support, many doors will be opened.

Don't do it all alone. Some people work great by themselves. If you're one of those people, I'm not advocating that you totally change your style. What I am suggesting is that you stay connected with others doing similar work. Let them cheer you on and listen when you need to vent. Beyond that, if you choose to share the work with others, they can relieve you of some of the responsibilities. When you're feeling discouraged or overwhelmed, your partners can help to renew your faith in the project or take on some of your workload. If you're not convinced you should work with others, think about what might happen if you move away or your life develops complications that severely limit the time you have to give the health ministry. All your hard work fizzles out unless there are others committed to the project. So stay connected.

Stay connected with other congregations that have vibrant health ministries. You will gain so much from each other in terms of ideas and encouragement. When your spirits are waning, you might get new energy listening to their stories. They might know of a course you can take or a book you can read that will address your situation.

Network with health agencies. Whether you work with them or just use them as a referral or resource, what they contribute will maximize your efforts.

Focus on issues you strongly believe in. Maybe it's mental health, maybe it's advocating for disenfranchised people, maybe it's physical fitness. Occasionally it helps to remember bad experiences, like the shoddy care an aunt received. This memory could be all the motivation you need to see that it doesn't happen to someone else.

Allow yourself to take a break from a project or move on to something new. Since you're working with a health team, someone else can take over.

Recognize if your project is not doing well. Get the help you need or simply end it if necessary.

Nourish the health team. Take time out for celebrations. As a group, do something totally different and fun once in awhile. Laugh together. Pray together. Share joys and concerns. Play together. All of this will make your health team stronger.

Start small. Don't take on too much. There is always time to add.

GUARD AGAINST BURNOUT WITH EVALUATION

To avoid burnout, reevaluate your health team's activities on an annual or regular basis.

- What is it doing?
- What isn't it doing that maybe it could be doing?
- What needs to be altered?
- What are your dreams for the future?
- Have a yearly celebration.

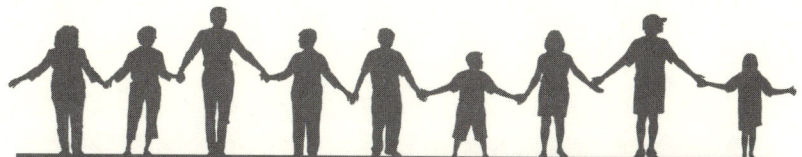

CHAPTER 6 SUMMARY

At this point, you have developed these four basic aspects with your health team: a purpose with a Scriptural, theological basis; team members and structure; goals and objectives leading to a plan of action; vision for the future. You are ready to take on your projects! You will become that guiding headlight that Martin Luther King, Jr. wants each of us to be.

Visibility and Communication with the Congregation. Throughout all of this, stay connected with your congregation: communicate! Keep them informed about your activities and initiatives. Invite continuing conversation.

Notes on Burnout. Perhaps most important of all: take care of yourself and celebrate your successes. Seek support, connection, and networking. Take breaks if you need them. Start small and realistic to be sure you can be successful.

PART 2
Resources for Your Health Team

Models of Ministry

Now that you've learned all the key components of building a great health team, here is a listing of health ministries in all shapes and forms. Your team and your ministry are unique to your context, so it will not look exactly the same as the models provided here. The following examples show the various creative formats of ministry that a health team can tackle. These models are a great source of inspiration and ideas for the focus of your health team.

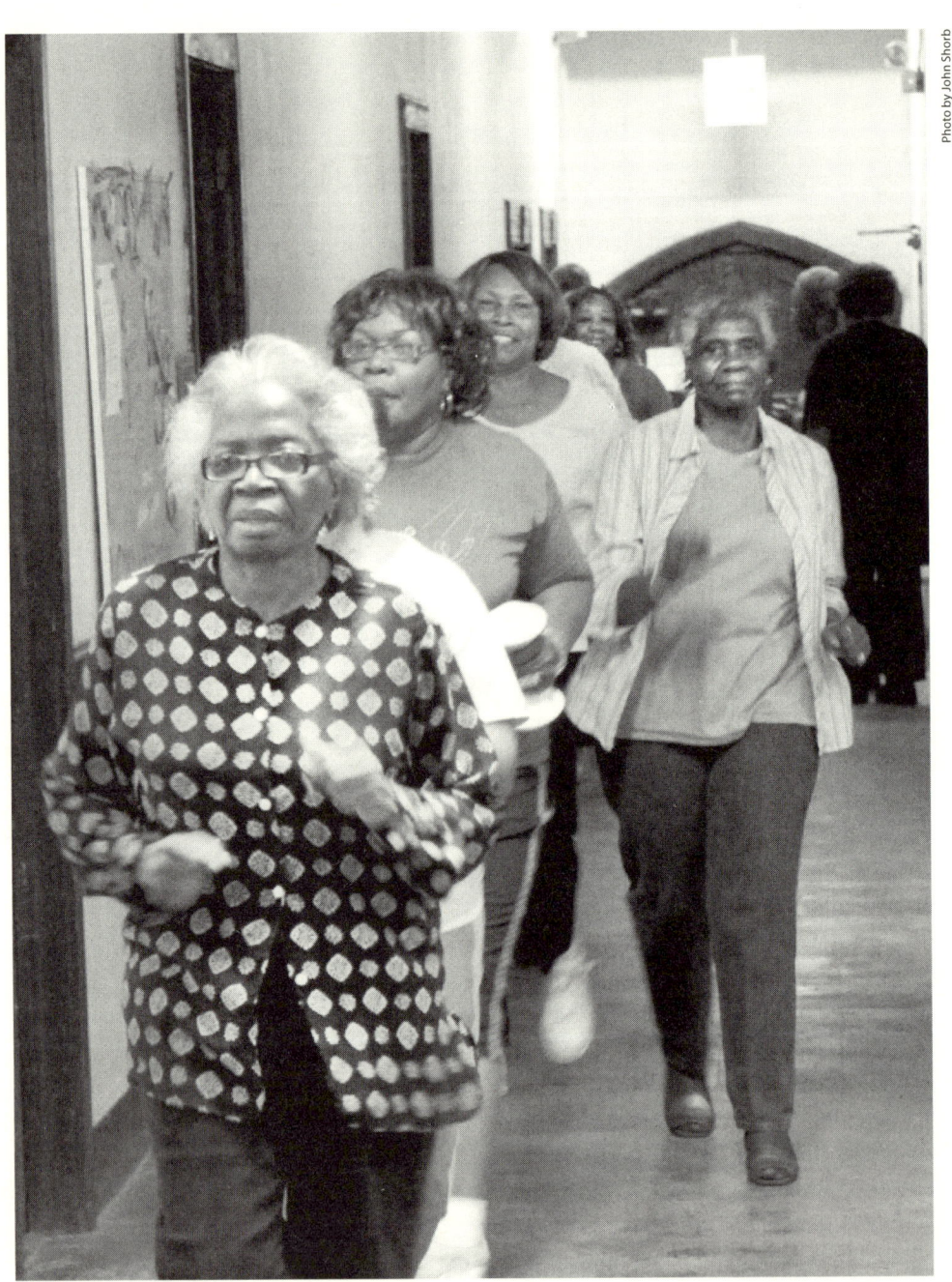

Every Tuesday and Thursday participants gather at First Presbyterian Church of Chicago for fellowship and exercise.

Community Walking Group

First Presbyterian Church in Chicago, IL
www.firstpreschicago.org

First Presbyterian Church of Chicago has a strong history of moving. Many of its members were leaders in the abolitionist movement, the temperance movement, and the civil rights movement. Now they are a part of the health ministry movement, and they are literally moving. Members and friends of the congregation meet on Saturday mornings to *Walk & Talk*. Using the curriculum developed by the Church Health Center, the group walks around their neighborhood and discusses Bible passages. In the late fall and winter, they use the aisles of the sanctuary as an indoor track!

For more information:
A Church on the Move by Reggie Weaver
published in *Church Health Reader*

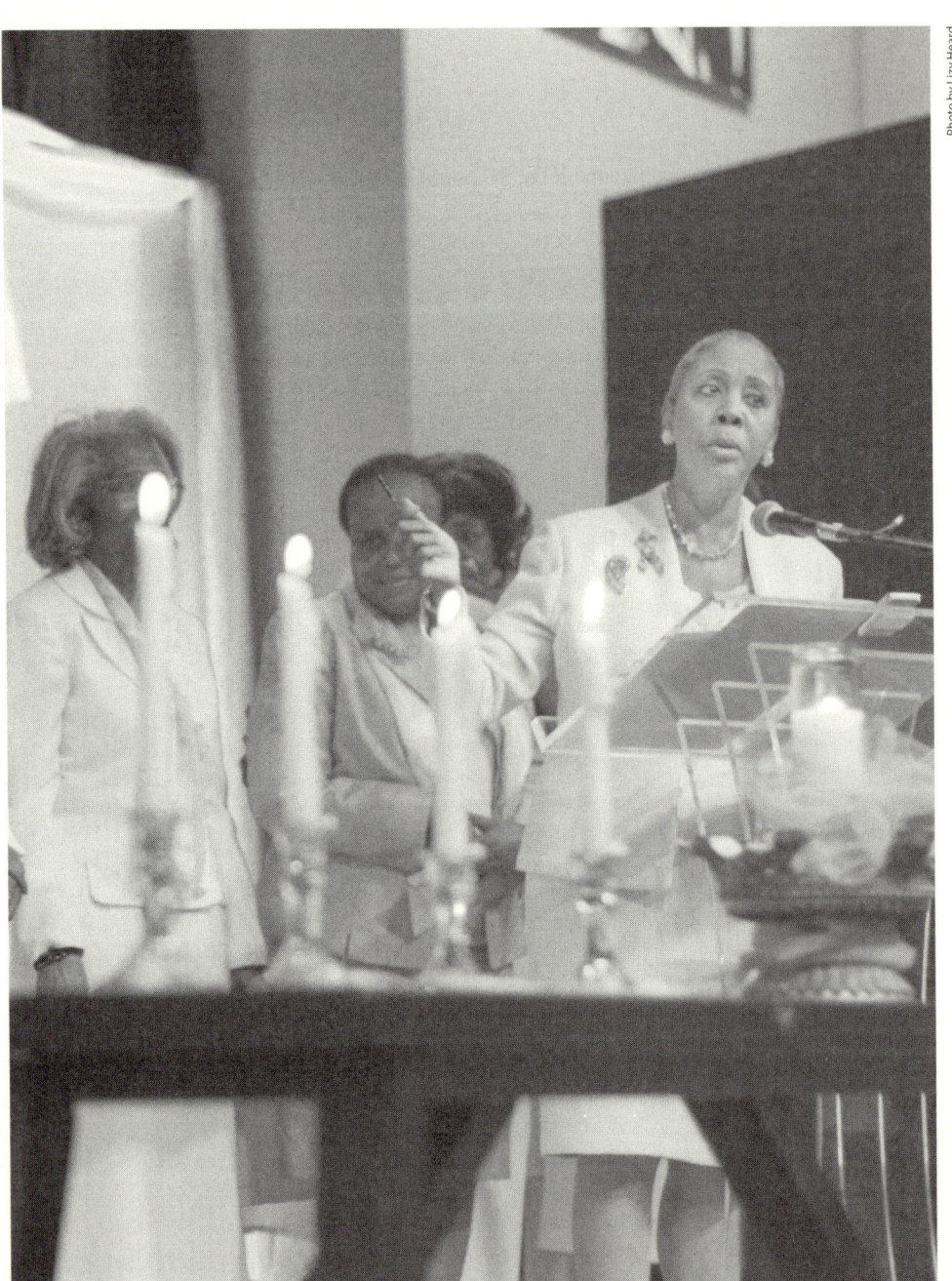

Photo by Lizy Heard

Gwendolyn Brown at the Carin' and Sharin' May celebration to honor women with cancer and those who support them.

Breast Cancer Support Group

Carin' and Sharin' in Memphis, TN
www.carinsharin.org

Gwendolyn Brown had a calling to support women with cancer, and in 1989 she organized the Carin' and Sharin' Breast Cancer Education and Support Group. Gwen and her volunteers provide financial assistance, community and—most important—a network of friendly faces to help address some of the issues of socioeconomically disadvantaged, inner city, African American women in the Memphis area. As she says, "Whether the journey takes you to hospice or to being disease-free, we will support you all the way."

For more information:
Carin' and Sharin' by Susan Martins Miller
published in *Church Health Reader*

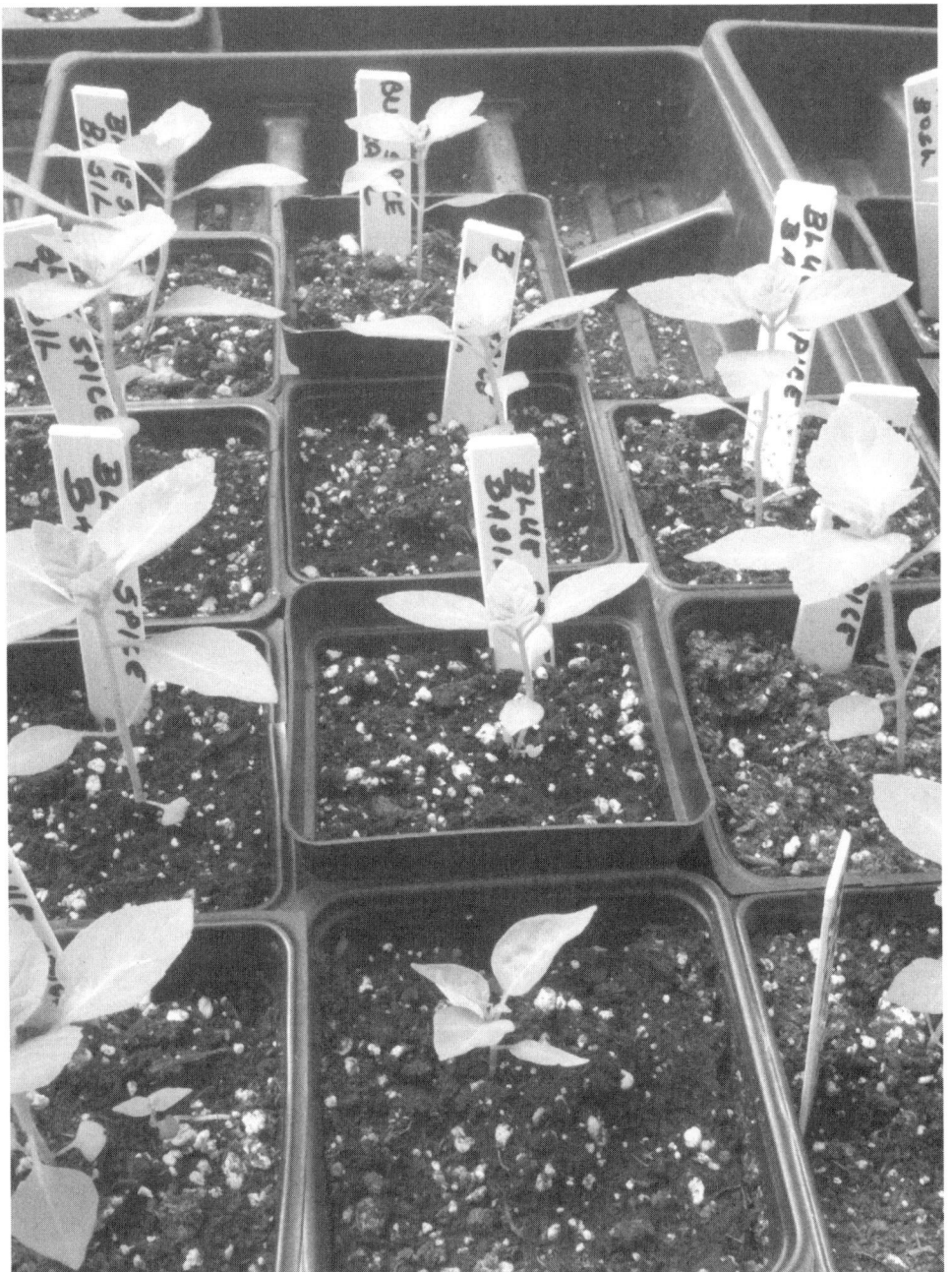

Plants for sale at Holy Comforter Episcopal Church.

Gardening and Mental Health

Holy Comforter Episcopal Church in Atlanta, GA
holycomforter.episcopalatlanta.org

Since the mid-nineties, about 70 percent of the worshippers at this mission church are people who live with a diagnosis of mental illness. They come from group homes for worship, community, and to work in the community garden. The garden is a source of healing and recovery for this at-risk population. They sell their produce at various community events. As their priest explains, "Gardening is a boost for their sense of what they can do. It creates opportunity for community, and it's very therapeutic." They even have their very own hot purple pepper, Holy Smoke!

For more information:
Holy Comfort: Gardening as a Means to Mental Health by Stacy Smith
published in *Church Health Reader*

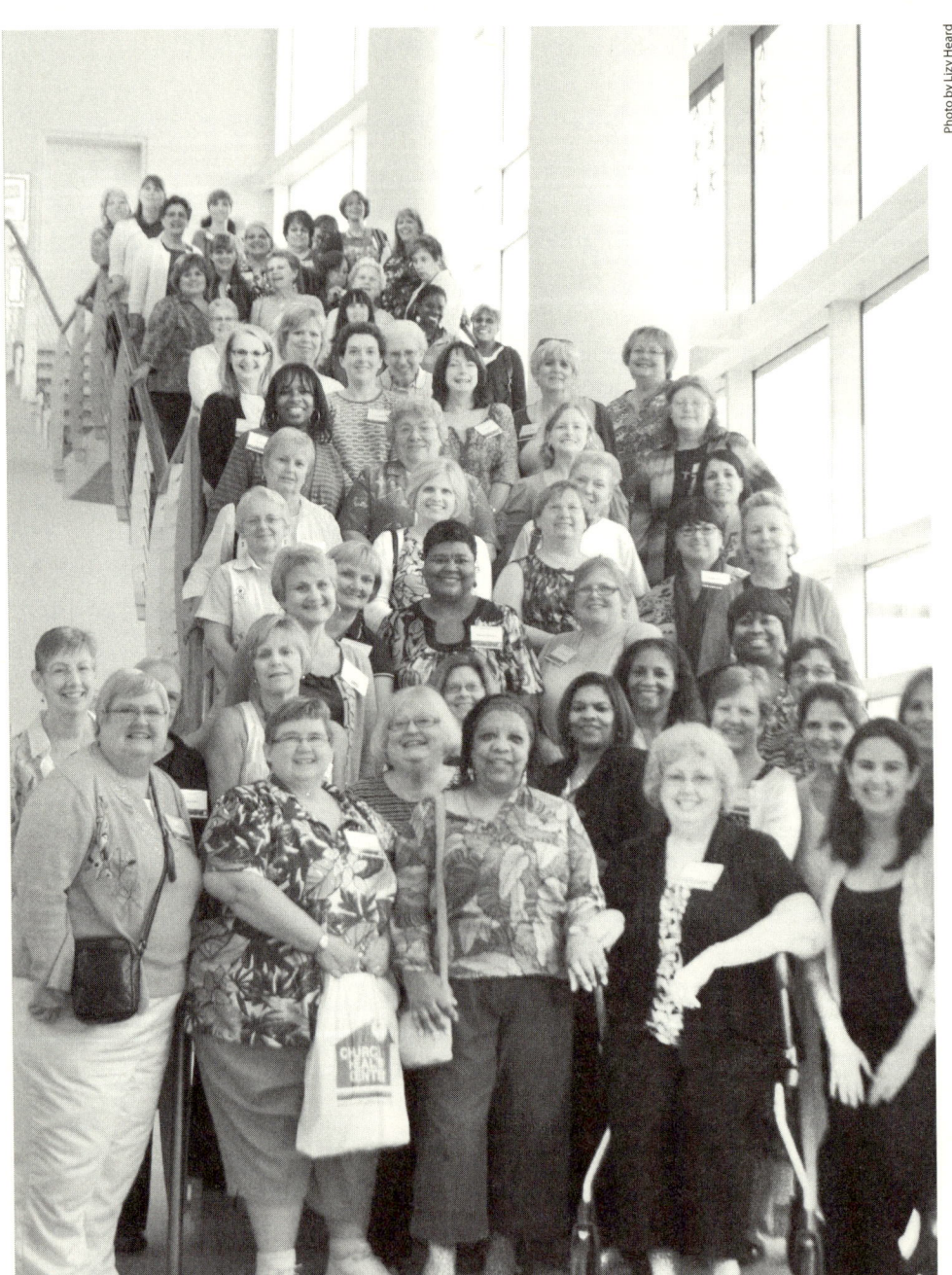

Faith community educators at Church Health Center.

Faith Community Nursing

A faith community nurse works within a congregation or community to better the health and wellness for all. To become a faith community nurse, you must be a registered nurse and take a course, most typically Foundations in Faith Community Nursing which is administered by the Church Health Center. *Parish nurse* was the first name for faith community nurses because the concept began in Christian congregations. When congregations outside of Christianity began adopting the model, the label gradually changed to faith community nursing. Your first contact for information should be the Church Health Center. They will have the most up-to-date information. They will also have a list of some of the faith community nurses nearest to you so that you can contact them directly. Since the role of every faith community nurse is different, be sure to talk with several and learn about a range of roles for the nurses.

For more information:
The Essential Parish Nurse, by Deborah L. Patterson

The Parish Nurse by Granger E. Westberg and Jill Westberg McNamara

Parish Nursing: Promoting Whole Person Health
Within Faith Communities
and
Parish Nursing: Development, Education, and Administration
both by Phyllis Ann Solari-Twadell and Mary Ann McDermott

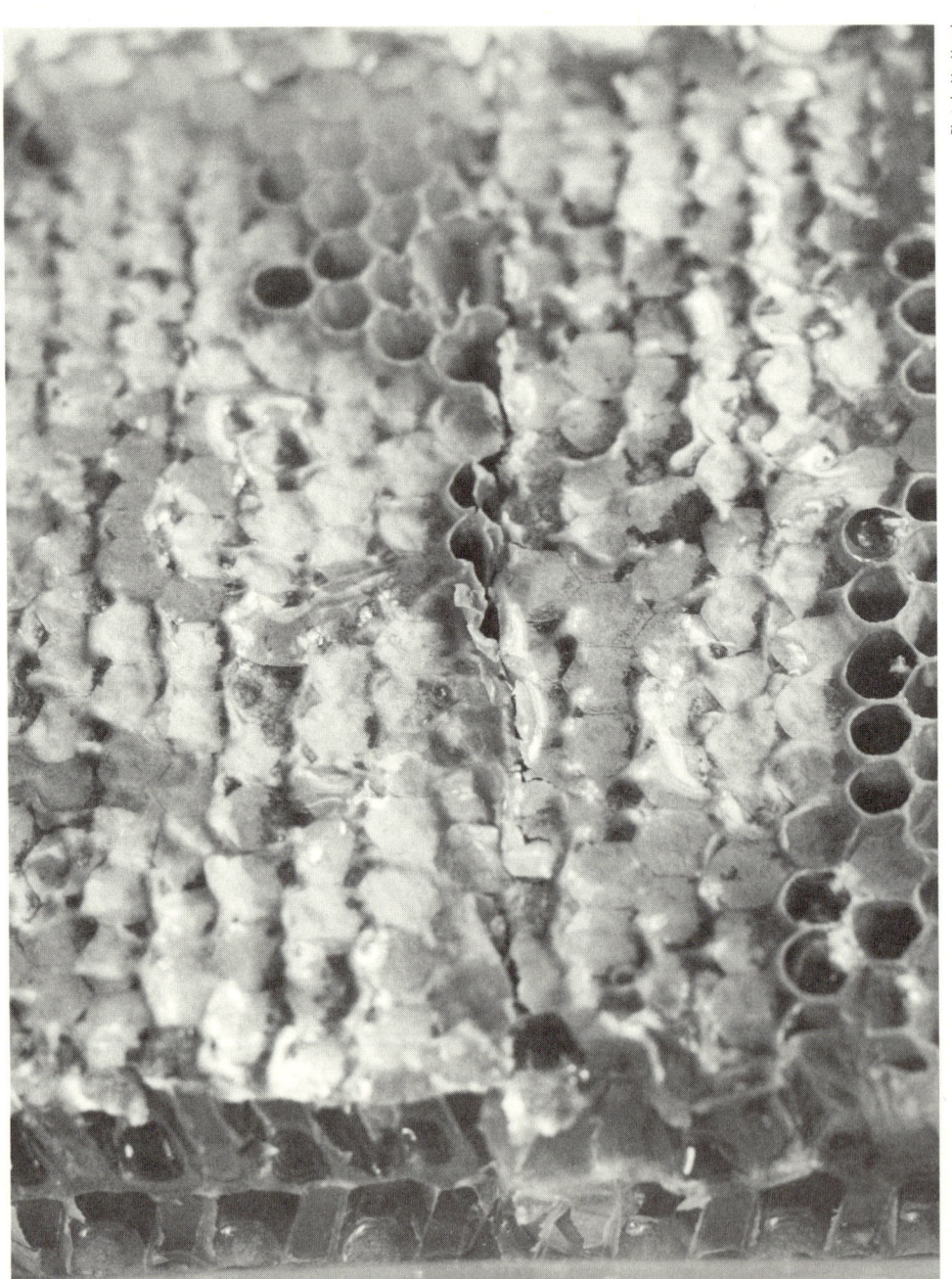

A honeybee ministry is a sweet way to promote health at your church.

A Buzzing Bee Ministry

Church of the Pilgrims in Washington, DC
www.churchoftheprilgrims.org

Over 40,000 honeybees call the Church of the Pilgrims their happy home. Through a partnership with DC Honeybees, church members created an apiary on their church grounds. As Rev. Ashley Goff says, "Won't they sting, swarm and create general havoc in Pilgrim's backyard? Just the opposite. Our buzzing, fat, furry companions keep to themselves as they are busy gathering nectar and building up their hives by creating beeswax, honey and honeycomb." They also help the gardens flourish, providing a healthy yield of tomatoes, eggplants and cucumbers for their Open Table community lunch.

For more information:
Ministry for the Bees (and us) by Ashley Goff
published in *Church Health Reader*

The gift of honey and the promise of God by Ashley Goff
published on www.faithandleadership.com

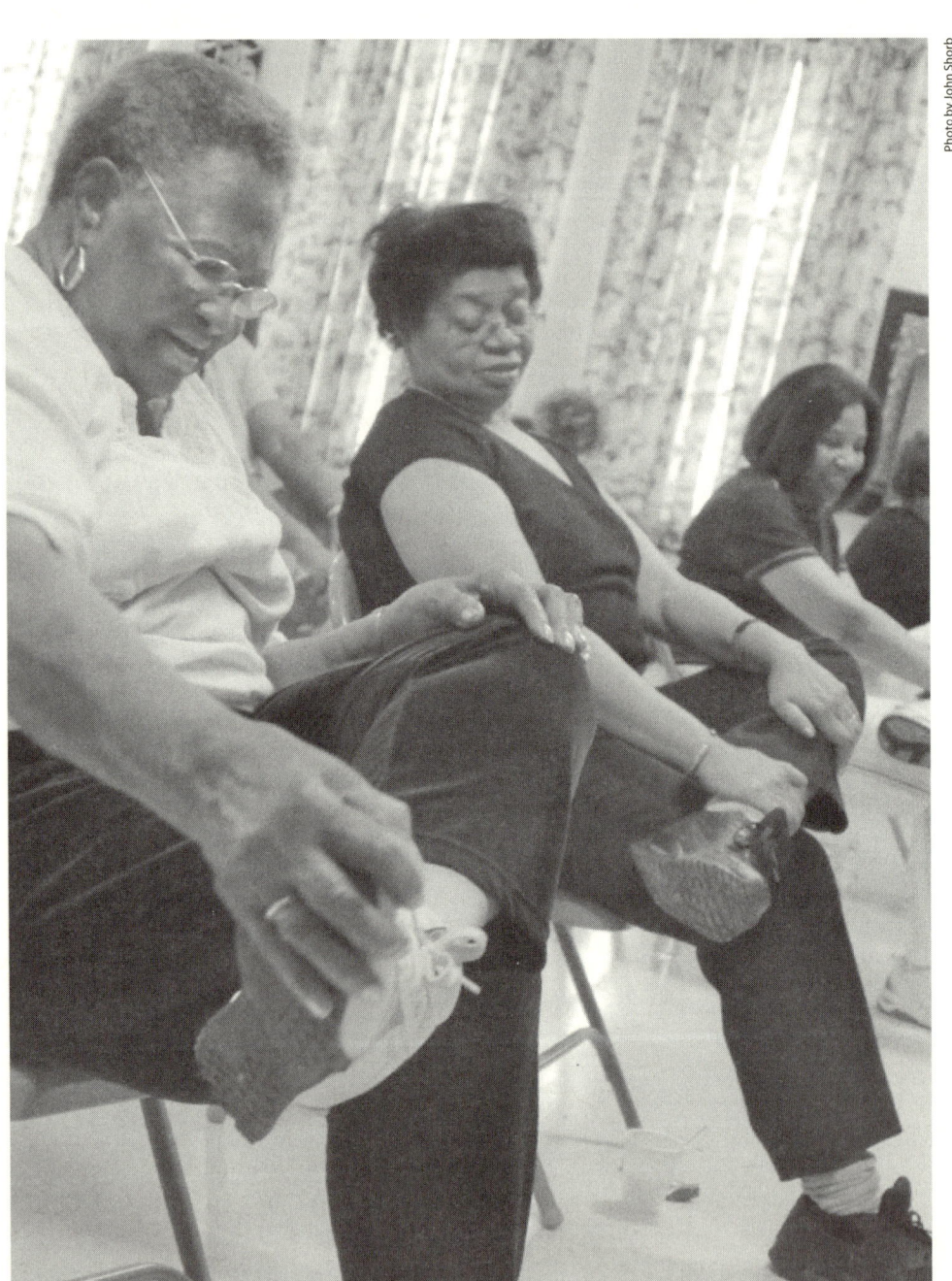

Participants stretching at the end of class.

Church Wellness Program

Trinity Lutheran Church in Monument, CO
www.trinety.org

Faith community nurse Jackie Sward began a health ministry at Trinity Lutheran Church with a grant of $400 and a team of like-minded people. She opted to use the Church Health Center's *Get My People Going! On the Journey to Wellness* curriculum to encourage whole-life health and held classes for participants on Sunday mornings. She also invited weekly speakers to discuss relevant topics and had a great turnout from her participants. As she said, the people who chose to commit to the class chose to make changes in their lives.

For more information:
Get Going! in the Spring 2013 issue of
Church Health Reader

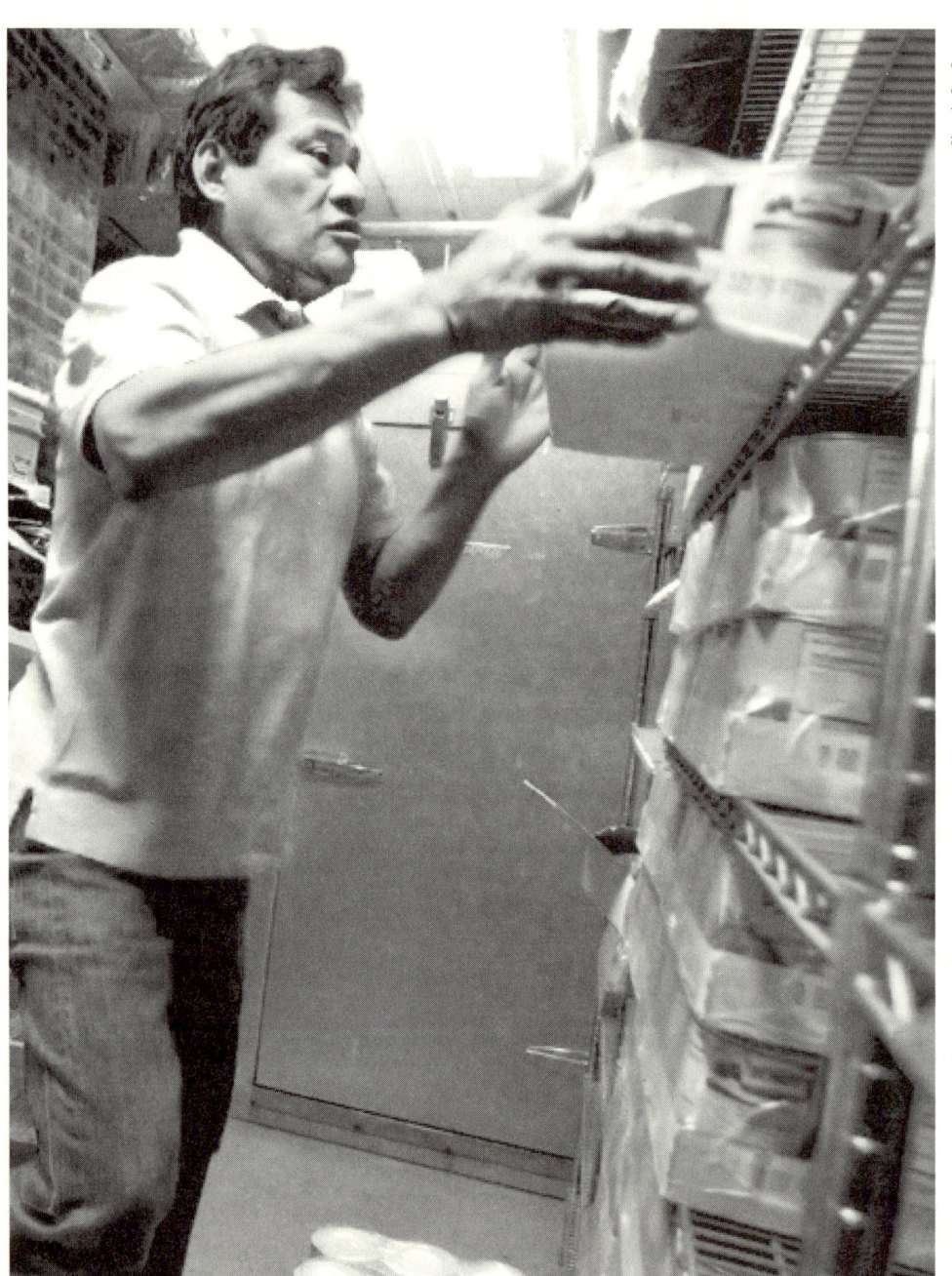

Shelves are stocked with a variety of foods to make healthy meals at WSCAH.

Supermarket-Style Food Pantry

The West Side Campaign Against Hunger in New York, NY
www.wscah.org

New York's largest emergency food pantry serves more than 40,000 families with enough food for one million healthy meals annually. But it's not the numbers that are the most impressive. The West Side Campaign Against Hunger (WSCAH) is an innovative, supermarket-style operation with customers choosing their own food, filling their shopping carts and "checking out" when they are finished. Customers are also invited to be part of the "Chef Training Program" where they learn cooking and food preparation skills. WSCAH changes the perception of hungry people by working in partnership with them, providing food with dignity and empowering customers to find solutions.

For more information:
Feeding the Whole Person by Barbara Wheeler
published in *Church Health Reader*

"A Veteran Chef Serves New Crowd: A Chef's Work With West Side Campaign Against Hunger" by Nancy Matsumoto
published in the *Wall Street Journal*

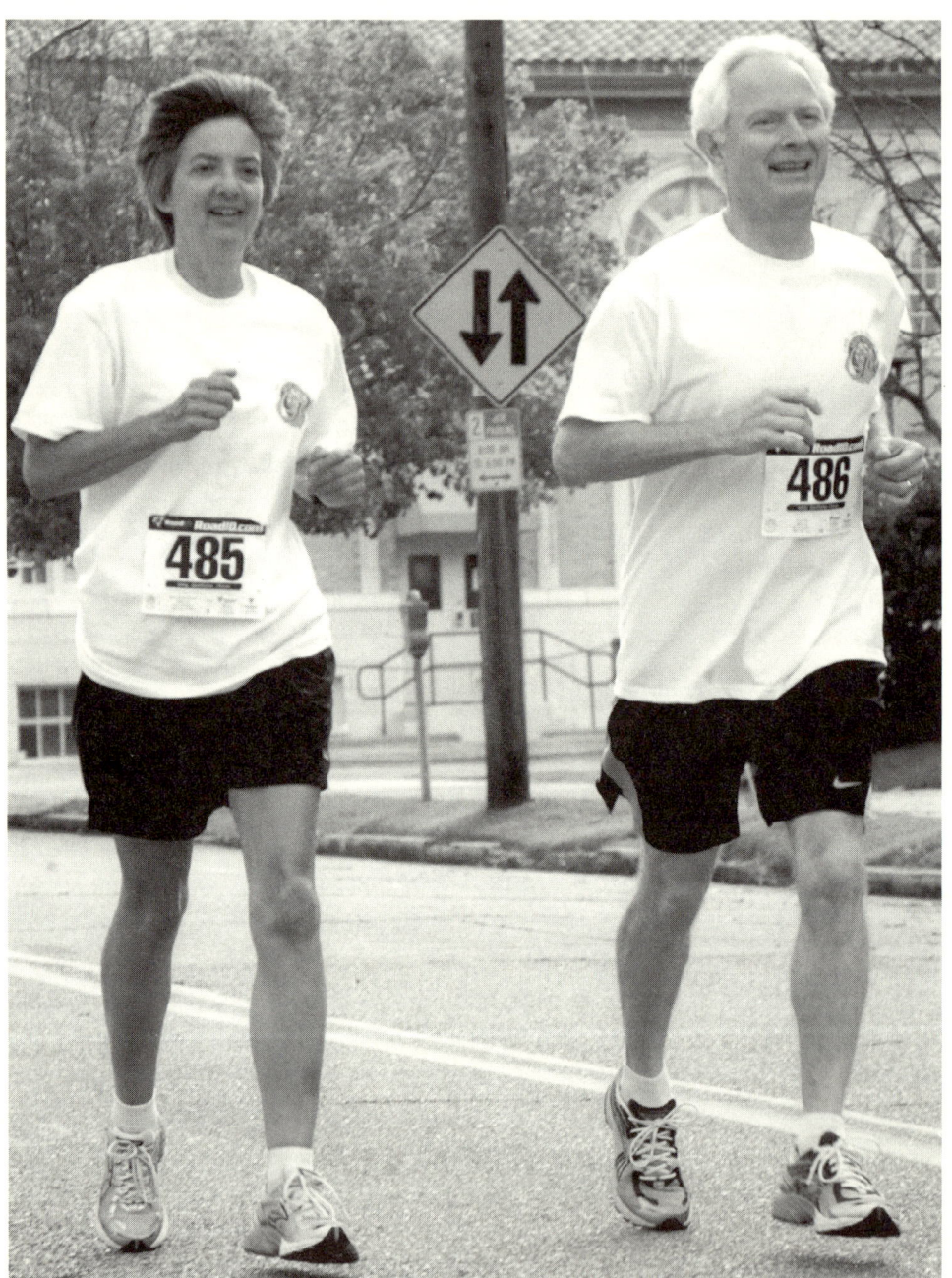

Bishop Hope Morgan Ward (left) and husband, Mike, participate in the Mississippi Conference's Annual Fun Run/Walk.

Clergy Health Competition

The Mississippi Conference of the United Methodist Church
www.mississippi-umc.org

In 2006, Lee Burdine introduced the Methodist clergy of Mississippi to a specialized pedometer system called the Amazing Pace. In the program, clergy wear pedometers and upload their steps directly to their computers. The Amazing Pace fueled some friendly competition among clergy to see who walks the furthest, and also made significant impact on health care costs. These changes in the clergy's attention to health care has impacted their congregations as people pay more attention to the improved health of their clergy.

For more information:
Clergy Health: A Priority in Mississippi by Darian Duckworth
published in *Church Health Reader*

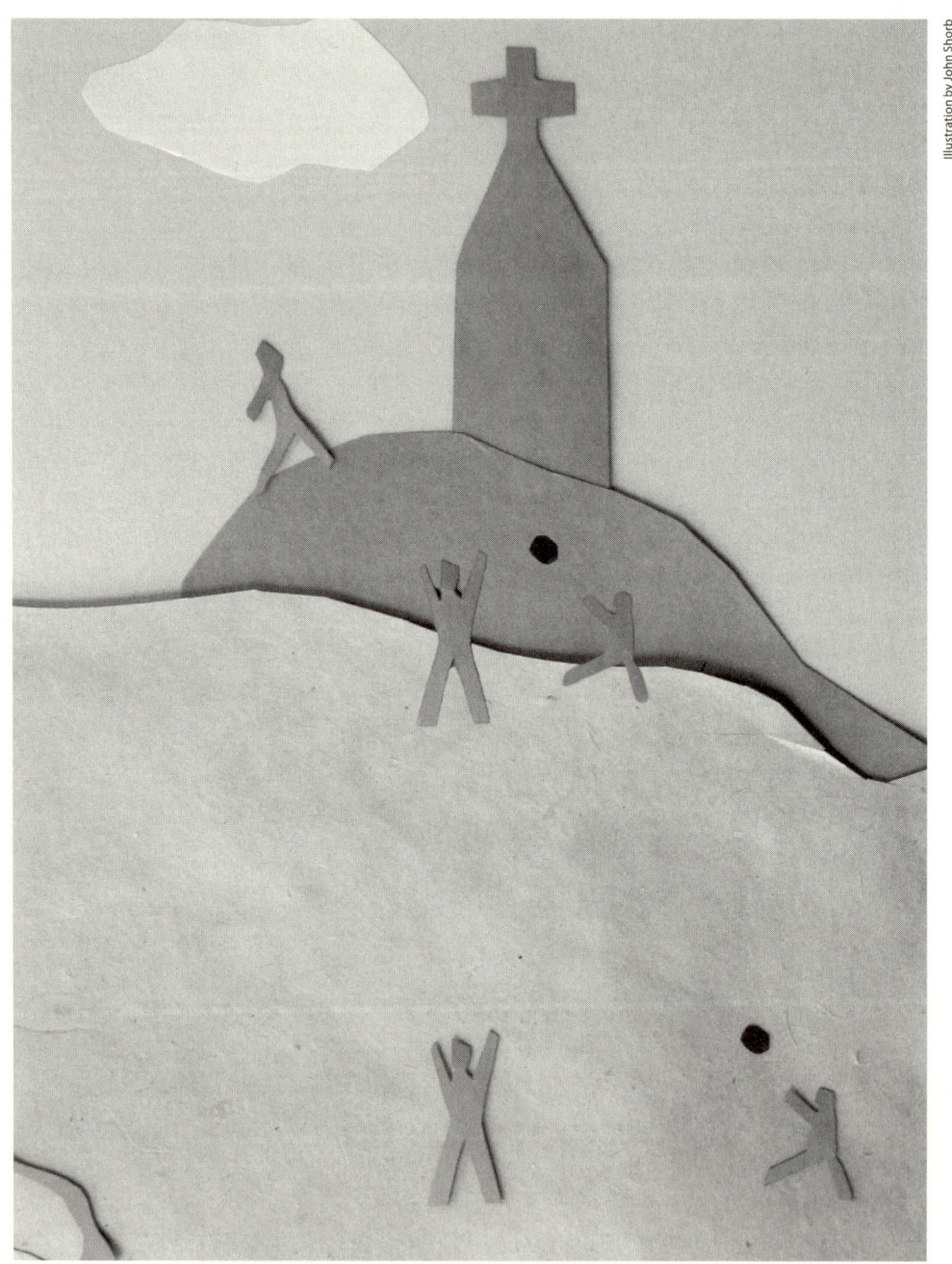

Enjoying the outdoors is an important part of the Shapin' Up curriculum.

Healthy Vacation Bible School

Shapin' Up Fitness Camp
www.kidzblitz.com

Michelle Romain developed Shapin' Up Fitness Camp as an alternative to Vacation Bible School to help kids have a passion to service God with their heart, mind and body. Shapin' Up is centered on 1 Corinthians 10:31: "Whatever you eat or drink, or whatever you do, do all to the glory of God." The camp is designed to teach children that they are created by God with a special purpose. Therefore, we need to take care of our bodies so that we can accomplish God's purpose for our lives.

For more information:
Shapin' Up: Michelle Romain discusses her Bible-based fitness camp for kids
by Sarah Ranson
published in *Church Health Reader*

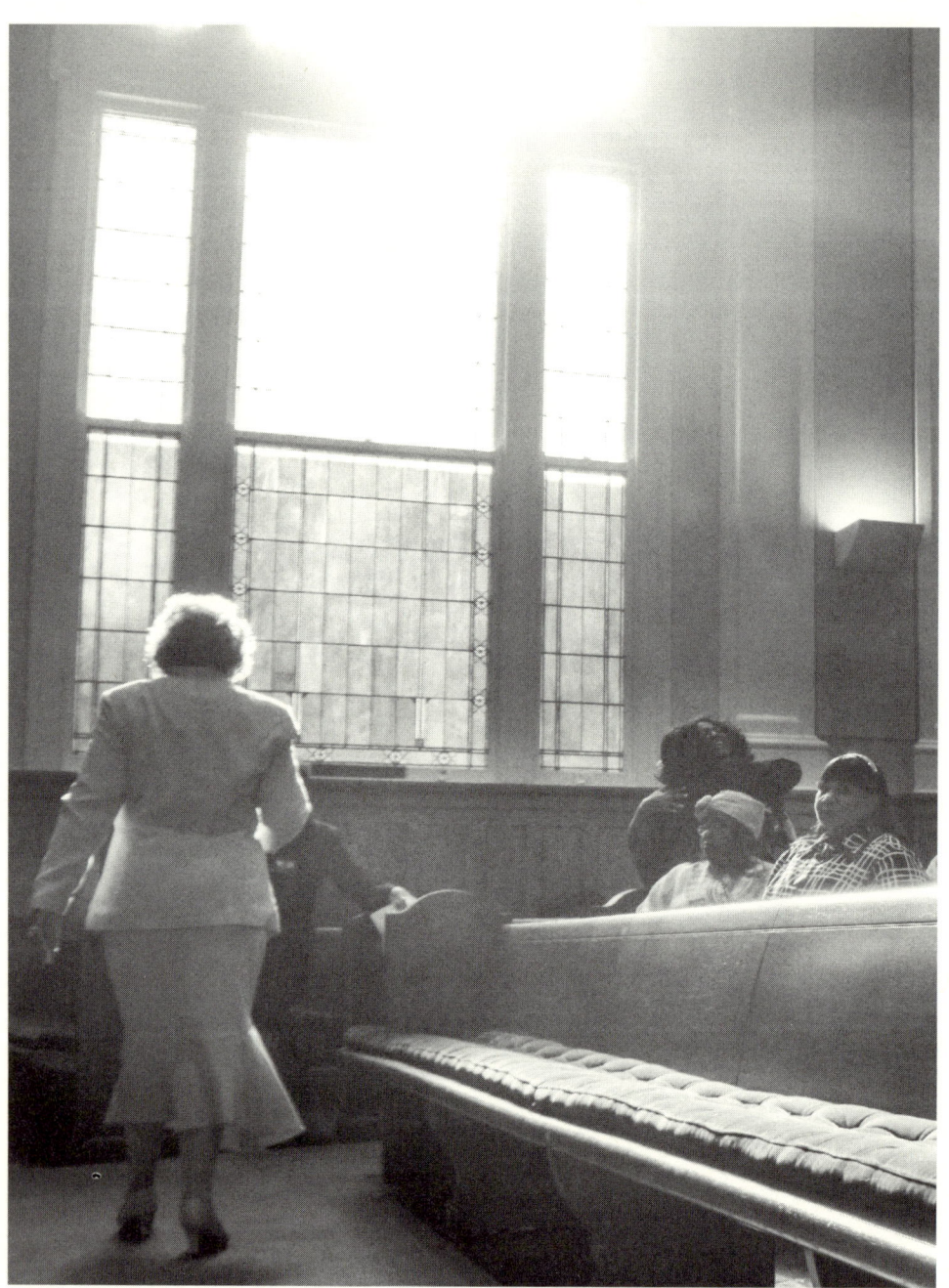

Members of the Ephraim Project at their commissioning service.

Congregationally-Based HIV/AIDS Advocacy

The Ephraim Project in Memphis, TN
www.churchhealthcenter.org

The Ephraim Project's name stems from Genesis 41:52 in which Joseph names his second son Ephraim because "God made me fruitful in the land of my affliction." The Ephraim Project, a special ministry of the Church Health Center's Congregational Health Promoters program, believes that people who are infected and affected by HIV/AIDS can be fruitful in the midst of their affliction as well. Congregational health promoters, or individuals who have been trained by the Church Health Center to serve as health advocates in their congregation, attend a specialized ministry on HIV/AIDS and become active, visual advocates for HIV/AIDS prevention and information in their congregation.

For more information:
Angels of Healing by Angela Dixon
published in *Church Health Reader*

Congregational Health Promoters by Kendra Hotz and Matt Mathews
published in the Spring 2012 issue of *Church Health Reader*

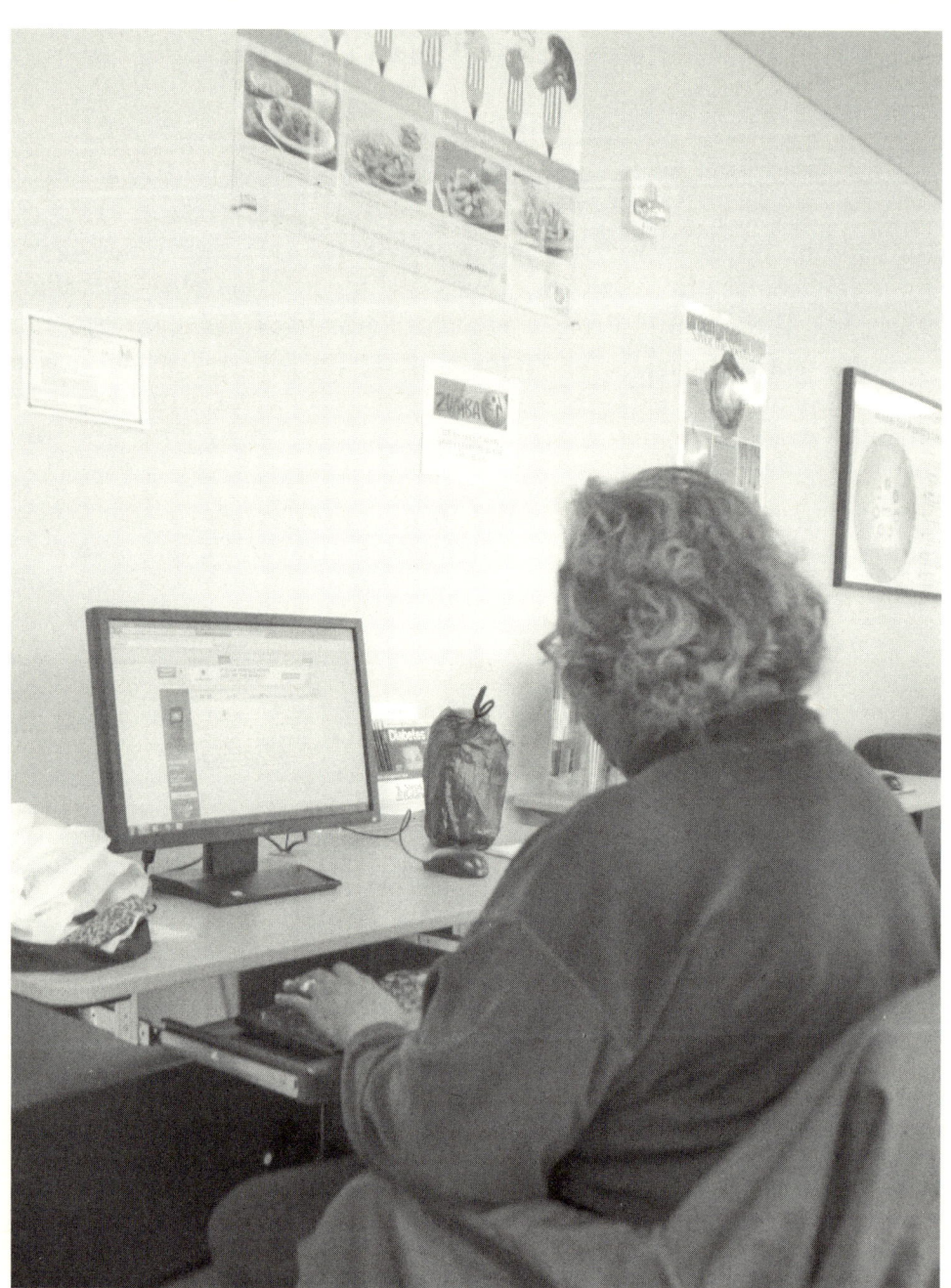

Computer skills provide self-sufficiency and assist with employment.

Job Skills Training

Old St. Joseph's Catholic Church in Philadelphia, PA
www.oldstjoseph.org

Founded in 1733, Old St. Joseph's Catholic Church is, well, old. But age has not stopped them from stepping squarely into the twenty-first century century. A distinctive element of their ministry is preparing people to enter or return to the workforce. The hands-on computer learning lab addresses the needs of individuals who cannot prepare a resume, navigate a job-search website or email a potential employer. In the process of the three-month course, participants create their own resume and practice filling out online applications for actual job openings.

For more information:
Job Skills for a Fresh Start in the Spring 2013 issue of
Church Health Reader

Key Scriptures on Health and Wellness

As we learned in Chapter 1, Scripture provides the foundation for many health ministry beginnings. We have compiled significant Bible passages, first from leaders and thinkers in health ministry, and then a listing of other key passages. As you begin your own ministry, take time to reflect on what each of these passages might tell you about the direction or core values of health ministry. Then you might brainstorm with your team or by yourself on which passages come to mind most readily for your ministry.

"Looking at health ministry in regards to scripture, the verse that has always resonated with me in scripture is a verse from Matthew 25: "And when was it that we saw you a stranger and welcomed you, or naked and gave you clothing? And when was it that we saw you sick or in prison and visited you?" And the king will answer them, 'Truly I tell you, just as you did it to one of the least of these who are members of my family, you did it to me.'" This has been a critical part of my thought process and why I think this ministry is so important. It brings a personal connection to those who need help, in addition to the actual services provided."
Matthew Ellis
CEO, National Episcopal Health Ministries

"Christ's ministry on earth was a healing ministry and our desire is to see the church live out that Christ-like model. We base a lot of our work on the John 10:10 passage, 'I have come so that you might live life to the full.' We talk a lot at Wheat Ridge about people experiencing fullness of life made possible in Christ."
Richard Herman
President, Wheat Ridge Ministries

"Health is a communal responsibility. We are responsible for those who may not have a voice. We are responsible for creating communities that enable people to be healthy. I see that speaking loudly in the Old Testament—particularly Isaiah 58 where it says that if you care for the poor, the widow,

and the orphan then your well being, your communal well being, your healing will be restored."
Mary Chase-Ziolek
Author of Health, Healing and Wholeness: Engaging Congregations in Ministries of Health

"In my service with Bon Secours, I assist in training, teaching, and mentoring over 144 people, affiliated with 106 congregations, to fulfill their call according to Luke 4:18–19, 'to preach the gospel to the poor, heal the brokenhearted, to preach deliverance to the captive, and recover sight to the blind, to set at liberty those that are bruised, and to preach the acceptable year of the Lord.'"
Sharon Jones
Community Benefit Ministry Manager, Bon Secours Virginia Health System

"One of my favorite passages is the story of the woman that bled for 12 years. Her faith was so great. She believed all she had to do was touch Jesus' robe, and she would be healed. We have a tradition of hope that if we work toward healing, that promise—that reconciliation—of a better way will be attained. This is how I see our healthcare system moving toward a place in our society where needs are met. That is a type of peace and hope where people do not have to make choices between medication or heat or water. The theological grounding here is this: the promise of people living fully human lives as God intended in creation."
Rev. Susan Friedl
National Council of Churches Health Task Force

These quotes first appeared in Church Health Reader's *Spring 2010 issue.*

Key Passages

In the beginning—there was health! The story of the Garden of Eden first shows us how God has created us to be healthy beings. We're not just body or just soul: the two are inextricably bound up in each other. As stated in *Dust and Breath* by Kendra G. Hotz and Matthew T. Mathews: "… as God's life-giving breath, soul permeates, saturates, and animates our body. We are ensouled flesh and enfleshed souls—whole selves whose spiritual identity and bodily identity are inextricably interwoven to form the singular fabric of who we are."[1]

Then the Lord God formed man from the dust of the ground, and breathed into his nostrils the breath of life; and the man became a living being.
Genesis 2:7

Next, God places Adam in a garden. God provided Adam with nutritious food (no Cheetos or PopTarts!), clean air and water and fertile soil. He was given all the resources he needed for a healthful life. God put Adam in the "garden of Eden to till it and keep it." Thus God provided Adam with meaningful work and opportunities.

And the Lord God planted a garden in Eden, in the east; and there he put the man whom he had formed. Out of the ground the Lord God made to grow every tree that is pleasant to the sight and good for food.
Genesis 2:8

God provides relationship. God also knew what people have recently documented in studies: that people are healthier when they are in relationships.

"It is not good that the man should be alone; I will make him a helper as his partner."
Genesis 2:18

God knows how to rest. A healthy lifestyle includes balance, a time for work and a time for play. This, of course, is echoed in the fourth commandment to remember the Sabbath day to keep it holy, but also in the very act of creating the world.

… and he rested on the seventh day from all the work that he had done.
Genesis 2:1–3

The Hebrew Scriptures show us how to be healthy in community. This includes being in right relationship (not only with God but also with others), living in harmony, working for social justice, caring for the environment, and making no distinction between body, mind and spirit.

Two are better than one, because they have a good reward for their toil. For if they fall, one will lift up the other; but woe to one who is alone and falls and does not have another to help.
Ecclesiastes 4:9–10

God's Shalom. Shalom means more than peace. According to Hotz and Mathews in *Dust and Breath*, "Shalom means the presence of all the conditions that allow every creature to flourish."[2] Shalom includes peace, prosperity, rest, safety, security, justice, happiness, health, welfare and wholeness. Wherever you see the word peace read shalom.

May the lord bless you and keep you … and give you peace.
Numbers 6:24–26

Wonderful, Counselor, Mighty God, Everlasting Father, the Prince of Peace.
Isaiah 9:6

As God's son, Jesus also provides healing. In addition to being a teacher or rabbi, Jesus was a healer in touch with both a physical and spiritual dimension of reality. Think about all the times Jesus comforted people, cured people, and restored people to their community and relationships. Jesus' ministry stressed healing the whole person: he did not separate the body from the mind and the spirit. Jesus dealt with relationships within people, between people and God, between people and their neighbors, and between people and the world.

> *And when they could not bring him to Jesus because of the crowd, they removed the roof above him; and after having dug through it, they let down the mat on which the paralytic lay. When Jesus saw their faith, he said to the paralytic, "Son, your sins are forgiven."*
> Mark 2:4–5

Jesus sent his disciples out to continue his ministry. He told them to preach the kingdom of God and heal the sick. Jesus wanted to bring people into relationship with God. To do this he used touching, speaking, commands, compassion and forgiveness. He also empowered his disciples and others to heal in his name.

> *John said to him, "Teacher, we saw someone casting out demons in your name, and we tried to stop him, because he was not following us."*
> *But Jesus said, "Do not stop him; for no one who does a deed of power in my name will be able soon afterward to speak evil of me.*
> *Whoever is not against us is for us.*
> Mark 9:38–40

The disciples continue healing after Jesus' death and resurrection. The book of Acts records how well the early church carried out this commission, caring for whole persons and not just souls or bodies.

> *But Peter said, I "have no silver or gold, but what I have I give you; in the name of Jesus Christ of Nazareth, stand up and walk." And he took him by the right hand and raised him up; and immediately his feet and ankles were made strong. Jumping up, he stood and began to walk, and he entered the temple with them, walking and leaping and praising God. All the people saw him walking and praising God, and they recognized him as the one who used to sit and ask for alms at the Beautiful Gate of the temple.*
> Acts 3:6–10

A History of Healing in Christianity

This timeline presents a brief history of healing within the Christian tradition with a focus on Western European and American histories. Christians had healing as a focus from their beginnings, even establishing the first hospitals. It is a history to build upon for our work today in health and wellness.

Early 2nd century
Christians develop church infrastructure to assist the sick. Deacons and deaconesses usually lead this work, which focuses on palliative care.

250–51
Devastating plague spreads throughout the Western Roman Empire, causing the church to expand its program of benevolence. The church at Rome is said to minister to 1,500 widows and others in need.

325
Council of Nicaea decrees that bishops are to start hospitals in every city where the church is established.

Mid-4th century
Basil of Caesarea builds his "New City" offering food to the poor and nursing to the sick. Basil's example inspires the founding of hospitals throughout the Eastern empire.

Early 5th century
Sampson the Hospitable devotes his life to helping the poor and treating the sick. With the help of Emperor Justinian he founds a hospital for the poor in Constantinople, which becomes the largest free clinic in the Byzantine Empire.

580
Bishop Masona of Merida orders that physicians and nurses bring all the city's sick, "slave or free, Christian or Jew," to the hospital and provide them with a bed and proper nourishment.

1191

Teutonic Order forms in the Holy Land as a brotherhood devoted to the service of the sick; later moves its base of operations to Germany.

Early 13th century

After being widowed at age 20, Elizabeth of Hungary gives her wealth to the poor and builds hospitals, nursing the sick herself.

1633

In response to the poverty endemic in France, Daughters of Charity forms to serve the poor and sick. The organization spreads to America in the 19th century and founds hospitals throughout the world. The Sisters contribute to the development of modern nursing.

1751

Dr. Thomas Bond and Benjamin Franklin found America's first hospital in Philadelphia "for the reception and cure of poor sick persons."

1765

John Wesley publishes the *Primitive Physic* in which he gave simple, practical advice such as eating a simple diet and getting fresh air. He emphasizes inward and outward health—nurturing our souls and bodies. He visits the sick in their homes and sets up a free church-based public dispensary.

19th century

The American hospital system develops through the stewardship of Christian denominations.

1905

Richard Cabot, MD at Massachusetts General and a Unitarian layman, realizes that patients had needs beyond their physical bodies. He helps create the first department of medical social work.

1913

Influenced by Jesus' teachings, medical missionary Albert Schweitzer establishes a hospital in Lambarene, Gabon, that grows to over 70 buildings, 350 beds, and a village of 200 people living with leprosy. He lives a life of service through the Christian labor of healing.

1924
Richard Cabot and Alfred Worcester, MD, conduct classroom courses for seminarians on topics like "visiting the sick," "caring for the dying and the bereaved," and "dealing with alcoholism and drug addition."

1930
Anton Boison, a pastor who struggled with lifelong mental illness, joins with others in forming the Council for the Clinical Training of Theological Students, which would expose students for extended periods to people suffering illness and crisis, mainly in mental hospitals. It is the foundation for clinical pastoral education (CPE).

1931
Helen Flander Dunbar becomes the director of the Joint Committee on Religion and Medicine of the Federal Council of Churches of Christ in America and the New York Academy of Medicine.

1944
Granger Westberg, a 34-year-old Lutheran pastor, becomes the chaplain of Augustana Lutheran Hospital in Chicago. This is where he began his work of bringing religion and medicine closer together.

1948
Mother Teresa begins her missionary work in Calcutta and ministers to the sick and dying. She founds hospices and homes for people with HIV/AIDS, leprosy, and tuberculosis.

1951
Granger Westberg moves to the University of Chicago where he is the first professor to have a chair in both the Divinity School and the Medical School. It was here that he wrote the best seller, *Good Grief*.

1973

Granger Westberg's first Wholistic Health Center opened in Hinsdale, Illinois. Twelve more followed in diverse settings.

1979

Scott Morris, a student at Yale Divinity School, visits Granger Westberg in Hinsdale, Illinois, to learn about church-based clinics.

1980

Five pilot health teams start in Chicago area churches. Evangelical Health Systems (now Advocate Health Care) hires Jill Westberg to promote health teams in churches.

1983

Granger Westberg pilots parish nursing Tucson, Arizona, and it is soon adopted by Lutheran General Hospital (now Advocate Health Care) in Park Ridge, Illinois.

1986

Advocate Health Care establishes the National Parish Nurse Resource Center (NPNRC) to share information about parish nursing and health ministry.

1987

Granger Westberg writes *The Parish Nurse* with Jill Westberg McNamara. Scott Morris founds the Church Health Center in Memphis, Tennessee.

1991

Rosemarie Matheus offers an eight-day program called the Wisconsin Model, the forerunner to the Foundations of Faith Community Nursing curriculum.

1997

The American Nursing Association recognizes parish nursing as a specialty practice focusing on spiritual care.

1998

Duke University Medical Center starts the Center for Spirituality, Theology and Health under the leadership of Harold Koenig, MD.

2002

The International Parish Nurse Resource Center moves to the Deaconess Foundation in St. Louis, Missouri.

2004

The International Parish Nurse Resource Center World Forum begins with 22 members representing Australia, Great Britain, Canada, Swaziland and the US, and contacts from South Korea also involved.

2009

World Council of Churches urges all member countries participating in the World Health Assembly to ensure that health care is free at the point of access for all, with a focus on equitable access for the poor.

2011

25th Annual Westberg Parish Nurse Symposium is held.
The IPNRC transfers from the Deaconess Foundation in St. Louis, Missouri, to the Church Health Center in Memphis, Tennessee.

2013

Paul Farmer, founder of Partners in Health, publishes *In the Company of the Poor* with Fr. Gustavo Gutierrez, a founder of liberation theology, on social justice medicine.

Acknowledgements

I believe this is the fifth revised edition of this book since 1981. This time around there are major differences because I worked with a team. Imagine that! In past editions, I had people who cheered me on, did some copy editing, but did not have the time to help shape the book. It left those editions wanting. Because I'm now part of a team, we each contributed the gifts we had to offer and made a far more interesting book: one with more life and energy. This edition focuses more on the action of the health team than the philosophy behind it.

Not only did my teammates polish my writing, but they also added some of their own. They envisioned a look for the text that would make it easier to read, a style that allowed the reader to glance through, glean information and know which parts to read in depth. No longer does the reader have to wade through pages of text to find those paragraphs of interest. Because of the graphics, the information leaps out. So thank you to my team members at the Church Health Center: Rachel Davis, Lizy Heard, Susan Martins Miller, John Shorb, and Stacy Smith.

Notes

PREFACE
[1] Martin Luther King, Jr., *The Strength To Love* (Evanston: Harper and Row, 1963), p. 98.

INTRODUCTION
[1] In 1973, with a lot of help from the W.K. Kellogg Foundation and the University of Illinois, Granger Westberg set up a Wholistic Health Center in Hinsdale, Illinois. Over the course of several years about fifteen Centers started in a variety of settings. At each of these there was a team of pastoral counselor, nurse and doctor who were seen as equal members along with the patient. Ideally each patient's intake visit was with the entire team. They cared for the mind, body and spirit of each person. They not only looked at a person's weaknesses, but also at his/her strengths. Wholistic Health Centers also offered an educational component to encourage prevention.
[2] Episcopal News Service, "Martin Marty speaks at NEHM first meeting," August 22, 1996.

CHAPTER 1
[1] Phyllis L. Garlick, *Man's Search for Health: A study in the inter-relation of religion and medicine* (London: The Highway Press, 1952).
[2] Interview with Mary Chase–Ziolek in *Church Health Reader,* Spring 2010.
[3] Morris, G. Scott, *God, Health, and Happiness* (Uhrichsville, Ohio: Barbour Publishing, Inc., 2011), p. 56.
[4] Phyllis L. Garlick, *Man's Search for Health: A study in the inter-relation of religion and medicine* (London: The Highway Press, 1952).
[5] Coffin, William Sloane, *Credo* (Louisville: Westminster John Knox, 2004), p. 139.
[6] Hotz, Kendra G. and Matthew T. Mathews, *Dust and Breath: Faith, Health, and Why the Church Should Care about Both* (Grand Rapids: Eerdmanns, 2012), p. 15.
[7] National Research Council. *Improving Health in the Community: A Role for Performance Monitoring* (Washington, DC: The National Academies Press, 1997), p. 41.
[8] Hackman, J. Richard, *Leading Teams: Setting the Stage for Great Performances* (Cambridge: Harvard Business School Publishing Corporation, 2002), p. 41.
[9] Edmonson, Amy C., *Teaming: How Organizations Learn, Innovate, and Compete in the Knowledge Economy* (San Francisco: John Wiley & Sons, 2012), p. 13.

JILL'S STORY
[1] Taylor, Barbara Brown, *Gospel Medicine,* (Boston: Cowley Publications, 1995), p. 7.

CHAPTER 2
[1] Patterson, Deborah. *"Ask Deborah: Starting a Health Ministry"* in *Church Health Reader,* February 21, 2011.
[2] Carter, Jimmy, "Accepting our Responsibility," *Second Opinion,* 1990.

HENRY'S STORY
[1] Rev. Henry Fischer, "Ministry A Many Splendored Thing" Sermon given at the 18th Annual Westberg Symposium. St. Louis, MO, Sept. 29, 2004.
[2] Ibid. p. 7-8.

CHAPTER 3
[1] Gunderson, Gary, *Deeply Woven Roots: Improving the Quality of Life in your Community* (Minneapolis: Augsburg Fortress Publishers, 1997), p. xiii.

JESSE'S STORY
[1] Miller, Susan Martins, "Breaking Down Walls of Isolation: The Sharing Group," in *Church Health Reader*, winter 2012, p. 18-19.

CHAPTER 4
[1] Bonhoeffer, Dietrich, *Dietrich Bonhoeffer Works, Volume 5* (Minneapolis: Augsburg Fortress Publishers, 2005), p. 84.
[2] Ibid.

KEY PASSAGES
[1] Hotz, Kendra G. and Matthew T. Mathews, *Dust and Breath: Faith, Health, and Why the Church Should Care about Both* (Grand Rapids: Eerdmanns, 2012), p. 3.
[2] Ibid. p. 86.

DEBORAH PATTERSON KNOWS HEALTH MINISTRY.

In *Health Ministry Advice for Everyone*, she answers some of the most pressing or perplexing questions on health and wellness in congregations. This book provides in-depth advice from healthier coffee hours to walking programs to caregiver support.

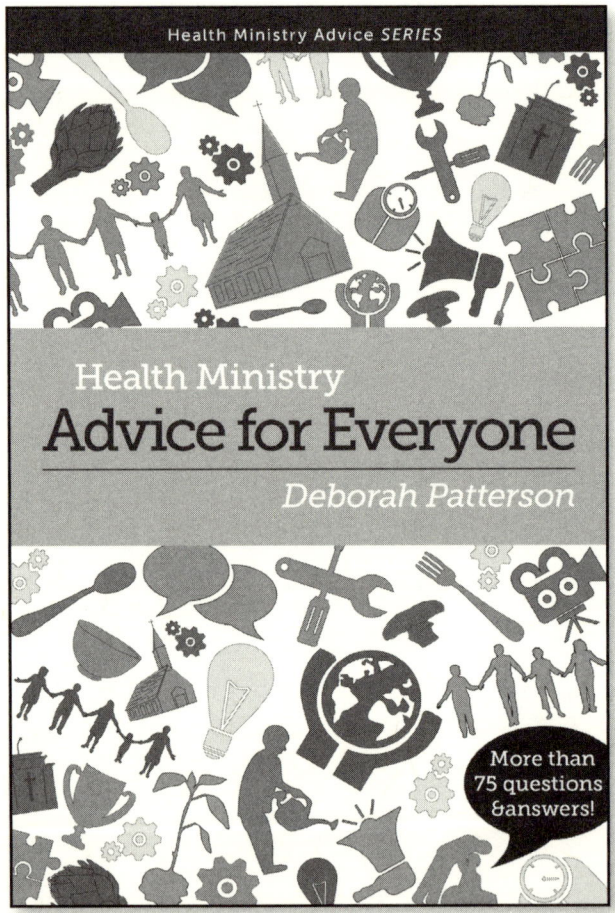

More than 75 questions & answers!
TOPICS INCLUDE
Children's Health • Mental Health • Clergy Health • $15 Coffee Hour
Healthy Food Pantry • Quilting • Caregiver Support • Walking Program
Starting a Health Ministry • Health Concerns in Worship

www.ChurchHealthCenter.org/Store